# An Age Old Problem

## A review of the care received by elderly patients undergoing surgery

A report by the National Confidential Enquiry into Patient Outcome and Death (2010)

Written by:

K Wilkinson FRCA FRCPCH - NCEPOD Clinical Co-ordinator (Anaesthetics)
Norfolk and Norwich University Hospitals NHS Foundation Trust

I C Martin LLM FRCS FDSRCS - NCEPOD Clinical Co-ordinator (Surgery)
City Hospitals Sunderland NHS Foundation Trust

M J Gough ChM FRCS - NCEPOD Clinical Co-ordinator (Surgery)
The Leeds Teaching Hospitals NHS Trust

J A D Stewart LLM MB ChB FRCP - NCEPOD Clinical Co-ordinator (Medicine)
University Hospitals of Leicester NHS Trust

S B Lucas FRCP FRCPath - NCEPOD Clinical Co-ordinator (Pathology)
Guy's and St Thomas' NHS Foundation Trust

H Freeth BSc (Hons) MSc RCG MSc - Clinical Researcher

B Bull BA (Hons) - Administration Officer

M Mason PhD - Chief Executive

The authors and Trustees of NCEPOD would particularly like to thank the NCEPOD staff for their work in collecting and analysing the data for this study: Robert Alleway, Sabah Mayet, Kathryn Kelly, Dolores Jarman, Waqaar Majid, Eva Nwosu, Karen Protopapa, Hannah Shotton and Neil Smith.

Special thanks are given to Professor Martin Utley from the Clinical Operational Research Unit at University College

# Contents

Acknowledgements 3

Foreword 5

Principal recommendations 9

Introduction 11

1 – Method and data returns 13

2 – Hospital facilities 21

3 – Patient comorbidities 27

4 – Pre-operative care 43

5 – Intra-operative care 69

6 – Post operative care 81

7 – Summary 97

7.1 – Care of fractured neck of femur 99

7.2 – Care of the acute abdomen 113

8 – Pathology 129

Appendices 133

Principal recommendations from *Adding Insult to Injury* 133
Glossary 134
Role and structure of NCEPOD 135
Hospital participation 138

# Acknowledgements

This report, published by NCEPOD, could not have been achieved without the support of a wide range of individuals who have contributed to this study. Our particular thanks go to:

**The expert group who advised NCEPOD on what to assess during this study:**

| | |
|---|---|
| Audrey Brightwell | Patient Representative, Age Concern |
| Peter Crome | British Geriatrics Society |
| George Findlay | Consultant in Intensive Care Medicine and NCEPOD Clinical Coordinator |
| Alex Goodwin | Consultant Anaesthetist and NCEPOD Clinical Coordinator |
| Tim Hendra | Royal College of Physicians |
| Chris Heneghan | Royal College of Anaesthetists |
| Tom Kirkwood | Institute for Ageing and Health |
| Thomas Lennard | Royal College of Surgeons of England |
| David Marsh | British Orthopaedic Association |
| Maura McElligott | Royal College of Nursing |
| Andrew Severn | Age Anaesthesia Association |

**The Advisors who peer reviewed the cases:**

| | |
|---|---|
| Robert Banks | Consultant Oral and Facial Surgeon |
| Rachel Binks | Consultant Nurse, Critical Care |
| Daniele Bryden | Consultant in Intensive Care Medicine & Anaesthesia |
| Helen Cattermole | Consultant Trauma and Orthopaedic Surgeon |
| James Clarke | Consultant General and Vascular Surgeon |
| Maurice Cohen | Consultant Geriatric Physician |
| Jeremy Corfe | Consultant Anaesthetist |
| Jugdeep Dhesi | Consultant Physician |
| Patrick Dill-Russell | Consultant Anaesthetist |
| Gemma Ellis | Consultant Nurse, Critical Care |
| Peter Evans | Consultant Anaesthetist and Intensive Care Medicine |
| Paul Farquhar-Smith | Consultant Anaesthetist, Pain and Intensive Care Medicine |
| Les Gemmell | Consultant Anaesthetist |
| John Griffith | Consultant General and Colorectal Surgeon |
| Richard Griffiths | Consultant Anaesthetist |
| Chris Hingston | Specialist Registrar Intensive Care Medicine |
| Tim Hodgson | Consultant Interventional Neuroradiologist |
| David Jones | Consultant General and Colorectal Surgeon |
| Cyrus Kerewala | Consultant Maxillofacial Surgeon |
| Richard Kerr | Consultant Neurosurgeon |
| Joerg Keuhen | Consultant Anaesthetist |
| Neil Kitchen | Consultant Neurosurgeon |

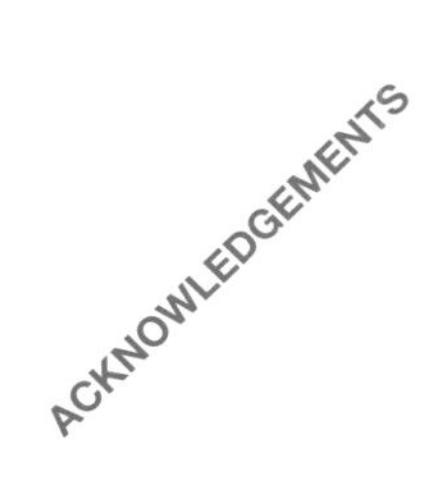



|  |  |
| --- | --- |
| Derek Kramer | Consultant Trauma and Orthopaedic Surgeon |
| James Manson | Consultant Surgeon |
| Colette Marshall | Consultant General and Vascular Surgeon |
| Sharon Mooney | Consultant Nurse, Critical Care |
| Ruth Murphy | Specialist Registrar in Anaesthetics and Intensive Care Medicine |
| Dave Murray | Consultant Anaesthetist |
| George Noble | Consultant, General Medicine and Care of the Elderly |
| Adam Pichel | Consultant Anaesthetist |
| Vino Ramachandra | Consultant Anaesthetist |
| Platon Razis | Consultant Anaesthetist |
| Alison Rawle | Consultant Nurse, Critical Care |
| Natasha Robinson | Consultant Anaesthetist |
| Neil Rothwell | Consultant Urologist |
| Prakash Rudra | Consultant Physician |
| David Saunders | Consultant Anaesthetist |
| Mike Saunders | Consultant Surgeon |
| David Seddon | Consultant Physician (Healthcare for the Elderly, General and Stroke) |
| Edward Seward | Consultant Gastroenterologist |
| Anne Scase | Consultant Anaesthetist |
| Craig Stenhouse | Consultant in Critical Care Medicine |
| Anne Stotter | Consultant Breast Surgeon |
| Jonathan Tilsed | Director, Acute Surgical Unit |
| Susan Underwood | Consultant Anaesthetist |
| Linda Walker | Senior Nurse, Operating Theatres |
| Neil Walton | Consultant Trauma and Orthopaedic Surgeon |
| Richard Ward | Consultant Vascular and General Surgeon |
| Barrie White | Consultant Neurosurgeon |
| Andrew Wyman | Consultant Upper Gastrointestinal Surgeon |

# Foreword

This report makes depressing reading. Too often it suggests a pattern of "one size fits all medicine" being applied to a heterogenous population with varying needs and falling short in ways which are both predictable and preventable.

The thrust is encapsulated in the finding that only 36% of patients received care that our Advisors classed as good (Fig. 1.4). That does not mean that the care provided to that minority was exceptionally brilliant, merely that it was what the Advisors would accept as appropriate from themselves or their teams. Although these cases were selected from amongst those who died within 30 days of surgery, the picture that it portrays is unfortunate. The subject is a vital problem for our society because it describes problems that are going to become more prevalent as the population of people aged over 85 is predicted to double in the next 25 years. The findings of our Advisors should be required reading for NHS managers and others who have to plan to deal with more and more of these patients and to ensure that the NHS is responsive to their needs.

Before looking at the detail, we must acknowledge the scale of the challenge. It is well understood that the elderly tend to be more vulnerable and to suffer from more co-morbidities than younger patients. It is equally well known that they require a style of medicine that is correspondingly sensitive to many needs that may not be obvious when they enter hospital for surgical procedures. The trouble is that our Advisors found that far too many of this group were not getting that pattern of care. It is also striking that even where there are well established and simple aims for good practice, these were often not being met. For example the National Service Framework for older people says that fractured neck of femur should be treated within 24 hours of admission provided the patient is otherwise fit for surgery. Obviously some cases have to be stabilised pre-operatively and theatre space may not be available, but it is deeply disappointing that in so many of these cases our Advisors found the target was not met. In 28% they thought that the operation was not performed in a timely manner (Table 7.1.7).

Speed is not the only consideration because the elderly lady who has fallen down and broken her hip may well have other problems that must be addressed before she can safely undergo surgery. She is more likely to be dehydrated, to have nutritional problems and to be at greater risk of thrombotic complications than a younger patient. She will be at risk of hypothermia, delayed tissue healing and skin viability will be an issue. The Service must respond to all of these needs if she is to recover safely from her fracture. She is also more likely to be confused and to have difficulty understanding the implications of the proposed surgery that should be explained when seeking her informed consent to the operation. All these issues are shown by this Report to have given rise to difficulties in this cohort of patients. Part of the problem may be that the young surgeon often does not require any help in diagnosing the lesion that has brought her to hospital – indeed it may be obvious from the foot of the bed. This does not diminish the need for all such patients to be seen by a Consultant within 12 hours of admission, because someone with experience of the other potential problems should be involved in setting the course from the outset (Table 4.4).

This need for consultant assessment of all acute admissions within 12 hours of admission was identified by NCEPOD in number of recent reports. It was recognised first in our study of patients who died or were transferred to critical care within seven days of admission *Emergency Admissions*[1]; it was repeated in *Caring to the End*[2], which looked at a group of those who died

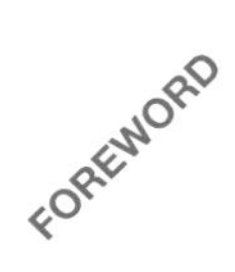


within four days of admission, and again in *Adding Insult to Injury*[3], which studied those whose admission was complicated by renal failure. Similar advice has been given by the Royal College of Physicians. It is unfortunate that in almost half the cases of patients treated for a fractured neck of femur no consultant review could be identified from the case notes at any stage between the admission to hospital of these complex patients and their death after surgery (Table 7.1.2).

The reader may wonder whether these people are being given the same priority as other vulnerable groups in society. Even though the accident that precipitated the hospital admission might suggest the need for reassurance about the patient's health and competence in other ways, less than a quarter were reviewed by a specialist in Medicine for the Care of Older People (MCOP) before discharge (see Table 2.11). Often part of the value of NCEPOD reports is to identify a problem and the importance of those who care for it, and to call for a wider awareness of their role. Our Advisors have pointed out that colleagues need to far more ready to involve MCOP physicians who may make a vital contribution to the care of these patients. One senses that the need for their involvement will always be more obvious in some cases than others, but questions should now be asked about the wisdom of performing surgery on the elderly at sites where these clinical teams are not available. Even patients whose problems appear straightforward to the team under whom they are admitted may have more complex needs than are recognised.

The chapter on fractured hips reveals an evident insensitivity to the concept that the bony injury may be the visible tip of a broader problem that needs to be addressed if the patient is to be restored to health and discharged home safely. However our Advisors found the same problems arose in many other areas of care. Again and again in this report one sees cases of patients who were cared for by doctors who may have been perfectly competent to manage the problem that they thought had been put in front of them, but were insufficiently trained to understand the subtle complexities that the case presented. As the broader clinical experience of individual doctors is replaced by more procedure-specific training, the authors suggest that this is a problem that should be met by more intensive consultant input at all stages of the patient pathway.

Our Advisors have said that a fully resourced Acute Pain Service is essential within the context of modern secondary care services, but they have found too little evidence that pain was being treated as the "fifth vital sign" and being monitored, let alone addressed and controlled. They have revealed what must sometimes be an organisational failure to respond to suffering since a quarter of these hospitals had no Acute Pain Service (Table 6.17) and those that did often lacked either specialist Pain Nurses or Consultants specialising in Pain Management. It is notable that these were particularly absent in the independent sector and this Report should serve as a wake up call to those responsible. People who are paying for their medical care are entitled to be as comfortable as those who are not.

One question that must present itself is whether the Advisors are being too harsh. There are three reasons for thinking that they are not:

1. The usual methodology that we follow sets out to guard against this. The clinical notes are not read in isolation, they are buttressed by a detailed questionnaire, which amounts to a commentary on the case by the responsible consultant. Both may only be read by one Advisor, but this happens in a supervised group setting and their opinions are discussed with their colleagues and one of our Clinical Co-ordinators who leads each group, before being summarised for the authors. If there is any doubt about whether the opinion reflects the mainstream view, or they are uncertain about their own view after discussing it with the rest of the group, the case is re-read by someone else.
2. The nature of the criticisms in most cases does not leave very much room for argument. Whether there is any evidence in the notes that a patient with complex needs was ever seen by a consultant is an objective fact.

3 The vignettes chosen to illustrate their points are telling, and in some cases shocking. These alone demonstrate the extent to which many of these patients received care that ought to be improved.

The second question is whether the numbers in each group of patients are too small to be a representative snapshot of the picture across the whole Service. There is more merit in this point and it must be recognised that we did not set out to judge the whole of health care in this country. Although we called for all cases within our category treated in the three months April to June 2008, we did have small numbers exemplifying some problems and as usual, some centres failed to participate properly. However the proposition that hospitals that fail to participate are doing things better remains counter-intuitive and there is nothing in this report to engender complacency. The page of shame, listing the centres that failed to respond appropriately is on page 146. We may hope that this will improve significantly now that the statutory Quality Accounts require Trusts to publish their participation, and our Local Reporters are being supported increasingly by our Ambassadors who will for example, help them to argue for more resources for copying notes.

The fact remains that this is an Observational Study, an assessment of about 800 cases of patients undergoing a variety of surgical procedures who died within 30 days of undergoing their surgical procedure. It is a biased sample in the sense that the majority of patients undergoing such surgery do not die during the following 30 days: our purpose is to identify points where there is room for improvement; to suggest how things could be done better, rather than to measure precisely how often the Service falls short.

Although these problems are complex and challenging, our Advisors have proposed a series of specific recommendations that could help to improve the situation. The Principal ones are summarised on pages 11. It is the role of NCEPOD to act as a ginger group: our Advisors identify shortcomings and suggest where and how things can be improved. Whilst we are not a regulator and it is for others to decide whether they need to act on our findings, it is our role to act as advocates – to disseminate the lessons of our study and to help professionals and managers up and down the country to recognise the relevance of our advice. This means that each launch of an NCEPOD report is but one step in campaign from when the Advisors recognise the Room for Improvement and the Health Services, as we must now call them, apply them to the care of patients. In this case this Report will be launched on 11th November when it will be publicised in the national press. Thereafter it will be available to download free of charge from our website http://www.ncepod.org.uk/reports.htm alongside all of the Reports NCEPOD has ever published. Then the work of dissemination begins. As usual, representatives of NCEPOD will be pleased to come to Trusts to present this data, to discuss the implications of our findings and our suggestions with those who are dealing at first hand with what everyone realises are extremely difficult clinical issues. I commend our Toolkit, which will enable people to replicate parts of this study within their own hospitals: again it will be there to be downloaded from the website. Junior doctors frequently find that using these Toolkits provides them with a worthwhile way of making a contribution to the improvement of the care of their patients - and moreover may develop into a useful publication.

Mr Bertie Leigh - Chair of NCEPOD

***References***


1. National Confidential Enquiry into Patient Outcome and Death. *Emergency admissions: A journey in the right direction?* 2007. NCEPOD, London.
2. National Confidential Enquiry into Patient Outcome and Death. *Caring to the End?* 2009. NCEPOD, London
3. National Confidential Enquiry into Patient Outcome and Death. *Acute Kidney Injury: Adding insult to injury.* 2009. NCEPOD, London

# Principal recommendations

### Chapter 2

Routine daily input from Medicine for the Care of Older People should be available to elderly patients undergoing surgery and is integral to inpatient care pathways in this population. (Trusts and Clinical directors)

### Chapter 3

Comorbidity, Disability and Frailty need to be clearly recognised as independent markers of risk in the elderly. This requires skill and multidisciplinary input including, early involvement of Medicine for the Care of Older People. (Clinical Directors)

### Chapter 4

Delays in surgery for the elderly are associated with poor outcome. They should be subject to regular and rigorous audit in all surgical specialities, and this should take place alongside identifiable agreed standards. (Clinical Directors)

All elderly surgical admissions should have a formal nutritional assessment during their admission so that malnutrition can be identified and treated. (Trusts, Hospital Nutrition Teams)

### Chapter 5

Temperature monitoring and management of hypothermia should be recorded in a nationally standardised anaesthetic record. This is particularly important in elderly patients. (Clinical Directors)

There should be clear strategies for the management of intra-operative low blood pressure in the elderly to avoid cardiac and renal complications. Non invasive measurement of cardiac output facilitates this during major surgery in the elderly. (Clinical Directors)

### Chapter 6

There is an ongoing need for provision of peri-operative level 2 and 3 care to support major surgery in the elderly, and particularly those with co-morbidity. For less major surgery extended recovery and high observation facilities in existing wards should be considered. (Commissioning Leads, Trusts, Clinical Directors)

Post operative acute kidney injury (AKI) is avoidable in the elderly and should not occur. There is a need for continuous postgraduate education of physicians, surgeons and anaesthetists around the assessment of risk factors for the development of AKI in the elderly surgical patient. (Postgraduate Deans, Medical Directors)

Pain is the 5th vital sign, and requires the same status as heart rate and blood pressure in the assessment and management of all patients. Clear and specific guidance on recognition and treatment of pain in the elderly should be widely available and incorporated into education programmes. (Postgraduate Deans, Trusts)

### Chapter 7.1

The British Orthopaedic Association and The British Geriatrics Society should provide more specific guidance on the ideal levels of seniority and speciality input into the assessment and decision making phase of the care pathway for patients with fractured neck of femur. (British Orthopaedic Association, British Geriatrics Society)

### Chapter 7.2

Greater vigilance is required when elderly patients with non-specific abdominal symptoms and signs (diarrhoea, vomiting, constipation, urinary tract infection) present to the Emergency Department. Such patients should be assessed by a doctor with sufficient experience and training to exclude significant surgical pathology. (Trusts, Clinical Directors)

# Introduction

The UK has a rapidly expanding population of elderly people. Currently one in five (12 million people) people are pensioners. At present there are approximately one and a quarter million people aged 85 or older. This group is predicted to double in the next 25 years and treble in the next 35.[1,2]

In 1999, NCEPOD published a report, *Extremes of Age*[3] and recommendations were made in this report around the care of the elderly surgical patient. The report emphasised the importance of team working, and the involvement of the appropriate level of clinician, in terms of seniority and experience, in the care of the patient. It highlighted the importance of post operative care, especially in terms of the availability of a high dependency unit. It was recommended there be sufficient, fully staffed daytime theatre and recovery facilities to ensure no elderly patient requiring an urgent operation waited more than 24 hours once fit for surgery. There was an identifiable need for specialised and experienced healthcare staff to ensure patients were receiving appropriate pain management.

The 2001 National Service Framework (NSF) for older people[4] recognised that care of the elderly in hospital is complex. It recommends that older people be given the early supervision and advice of a specialist team when admitted to an acute general hospital. In particular it stated that there should be involvement of a consultant in old age medicine or rehabilitation, so that appropriate treatment and management decisions are made. As well as medical consultants who care for the elderly, specialist nurses/nurse consultants, physiotherapists together with occupational therapists, speech and language specialists, dieticians, social workers and care managers; and pharmacists are required.

Recommendations extended to emergency care with a particular focus on transfer from the Emergency Department (ED) as soon as possible. Other common themes are attention to fluid balance, pain management, pressure sore risk management, falls and immobility, nutritional status and cognitive impairment. There is recognition that with advancing age there is an increased risk of post operative complications, which in part relates to a higher incidence of coexisting disease.

In relation to acute surgery, the NSF recommends that operations for fractured hip repair (which make up a large percentage of operations in the elderly) should be carried out within the first 24 hours of admission, and patients should be mobilised within the first 48 hours where appropriate. Discharge from hospital needs to be carefully planned with the full involvement of a multidisciplinary team, the family and carers.[4]

What are the main reasons for surgical admission? In 1997/98 NCEPOD[3] found that the most common operative procedures were hemiarthroplasty and sliding hip screw (24% and 23% respectively), laparotomy (13%) and amputation.

Falls represent half of hospital admissions for accidental injury and many of these are in the over 65 group and involve the femur.[5] We know that half of patients with a hip fracture never regain full mobility and one in three dies within three months. However, the recent Royal College of Physicians Falls Audit demonstrated that many patients with fractured neck of femur still took > 48 hours to reach the operating theatre.[6] It is very difficult to tell whether patients who wait > 24 hours for surgery do so because of inferior systems of care or because comorbidity precludes early surgery.[7,8]

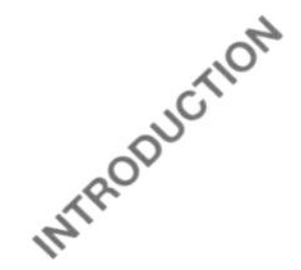


Future studies therefore need to try and identify whether patients wait > 24 hours when they have been declared fit and ready for surgery.

Laparotomy and bowel resection is one of the most commonly performed major operations in the elderly both in the elective and emergency setting. These patients may present for surgery with acute fluid and electrolyte imbalance due to the combined effects of inadequate intake relative to fluid loss, which may be superimposed on reduced renal reserve and (in the emergency setting) sepsis and third space losses. They require skilled resuscitation, careful peri-operative monitoring of cardiovascular parameters and fluid balance. This needs to commence preoperatively, and be continued into the intra-operative and post operative period.

In this study NCEPOD will review a sample of deaths following emergency and elective surgery in the elderly population.

***References***


1. Help the aged. *Facts and figures about older people in the UK. July 2008.* 2008. http://www.helptheaged.org.uk/NR/rdonlyres/318C26CA-F4EB-4A91-B77CA2867F85AF63/0/uk_facts.pdf

2. Office of National Statistics. *Population; Ageing.* 2008. http://www.statistics.gov.uk/cci/nugget.asp?id=949

3. National Confidential Enquiry into Patient Outcome and Death. *Extremes of Age, The 1999 report of the National Confidential Enquiry into Peri-operative Death.* 1999. NCEPOD, London

4. Department of Health. *The National Service Framework for older people.* 2001. Crown Copyright.

5. Battle A, Aylin P. Mortality associated with delay in operation after hip fracture – an observations study. *British Medical Journal*; 2006; 332, 947 - 951

6. Royal College of Physicians. *National Clinical Audit of Falls and Bone Health in older people.* 2007. Royal College of Physicians & Health Care Commission.

7. Bryson G. Waiting for hip fracture repair – Do outcomes and patients suffer? *Canadian Journal of Anaesthesiology,* 2008; 55(3), 135 - 139

8. Shiga T et al. Is operative delay associated with increased mortality of hip fracture patients? Systematic review meta-analysis and meta-regression. *Canadian Journal of Anaesthesiology,* 2008; 55(3), 146 - 154

# 1 – Method and data returns

## Aim

To explore remediable factors in the processes of care of patients aged 80 or older who died within 30 days of a surgical procedure.

## Objectives

The expert group identified objectives that would address the overall aim of the study and these will be explored throughout the following chapters:

- Fluid management
- The seniority of clinicians involved in intra-operative care
- Delays in surgery (due to scheduling, and the management of the patient's physical status)
- Anaesthetic management including pre-operative assessment
- Acute pain management
- Post operative cognitive dysfunction
- Use of critical care facilities
- Nutrition
- Comorbidities
- Medications including thromboembolism prophylaxis
- Consent
- Prevention of peri-operative hypothermia

## Expert group

A multidisciplinary group of experts comprising consultants from surgery, anaesthetics, medicine for the care of older people, (MCOP) trauma and orthopaedics, intensive care medicine, nursing, the Institute for Ageing and Health, a lay representative and a scientific advisor contributed to the design of the study and reviewed the findings.

## Population

All patients aged 80 and over who died within 30 days of a surgical procedure carried out between 1st April 2008 – 30th June 2008 were included in the study.

## Hospital participation

National Health Service hospitals in England, Wales and Northern Ireland were expected to participate, as well as hospitals in the independent sector and public hospitals in the Isle of Man, Guernsey and Jersey. Within each hospital, a named contact, referred to as the NCEPOD Local Reporter, acted as a link between NCEPOD and the hospital staff, facilitating case identification, dissemination of questionnaires and data collation.

## Exclusions

A number of Office of Population Censuses and Surveys (OPCS) classification of intervention and procedure codes were excluded where performed in isolation. Patients who were discharged alive from that episode of care, or who died more than 30 days following their surgical procedure were also excluded.

## Case ascertainment

Cases were identified using OPCS codes. The NCEPOD Local Reporter identified all patients who died within their hospital(s) during the study period, within 30 days of a surgical procedure (the first/primary surgical procedure of their final admission). The information requested for each case included the details of the surgeon and anaesthetist who carried out the procedure. All cases identified to NCEPOD with an included OPCS code were included in the study.

### Questionnaires and case notes

Three questionnaires were used to collect data for this study, one surgical questionnaire; one anaesthetic questionnaire where applicable; and one organisational questionnaire per site.

### Surgical questionnaire

The surgical questionnaire was sent to the surgeon who carried out the primary procedure of the final admission. This questionnaire covered all aspects of patient care from admission, to death. The number of questionnaires was not limited per surgeon. These questionnaires were either sent directly to the surgeon or via the local reporter for dissemination depending on the Trust.

### Anaesthetic questionnaire

The anaesthetic questionnaire was sent to the anaesthetist whose care the patient was under at the time of their procedure. This questionnaire covered all aspects of patient care from admission, to death, and again the number of questionnaires was not limited per anaesthetist. The anaesthetic questionnaire did not need to be completed where the operation was carried out under local anaesthetic. These questionnaires were either sent directly to the anaesthetist or via the local reporter for dissemination depending on the Trust.

### Organisational questionnaire

This questionnaire was used to collect data on a site by site basis so we were aware of the facilities available at each site for each patient in the study. Data collected concerned operating facilities, special care areas, pre- and post operative assessment facilities, and audit.

The organisational questionnaire was sent to the Local Reporter for completion in collaboration with the relevant specialties, and the Medical Director was also informed of this at the same time, and asked to contribute as appropriate.

### Case notes

For each case, the following case note extracts were requested to enable peer review:

- Pre-assessment clinic notes
- Transfer documentation
- Inpatient and outpatient annotations from pre-admission to death
- Integrated care pathways
- Nursing notes (including Waterlow, Mental State Examination records, Pain Assessment records, Nutrition Assessment records)
- Drug charts
- Imaging reports
- ICU charts
- Fluid balance charts
- Operation notes
- Notes from MDT meetings
- Consent forms
- Pathology results
- Haematology (FBC), biochemistry results (LFT, U&E), EDTA creatinine clearance
- End of Life Pathway documentation
- Incident report form and details of outcome
- Post mortem report
- Discharge summary

- Anaesthetic charts
- Pre-anaesthetic or pre-admission protocols/ checklists
- Recovery room records
- DNAR Report

These were anonymised on receipt at NCEPOD.

## Advisor groups

A multidisciplinary group of Advisors was recruited to review the case notes and associated questionnaires. The group of Advisors comprised clinicians from the following specialties: surgery (general and specialty), anaesthesia, medicine (general and the relevant specialties), Medicine for the Care of Older People (MCOP), Trauma and Orthopaedics (T&O), intensive care medicine, radiology and nursing.

All questionnaires and case notes were anonymised by the non-clinical staff at NCEPOD. All patient, clinician and hospital identifiers were removed. Neither clinical co-ordinators at NCEPOD, nor the Advisors had access to such identifiers.

Each case was reviewed by one advisor within a multidisciplinary group. At regular intervals throughout the meeting, the chair allowed a period of discussion for each advisor to summarise their cases and ask for opinions from other specialties or raise aspects of a case for discussion.

All data were analysed using Microsoft Access and Excel by the research staff at NCEPOD.

The findings of the report were reviewed by the Expert Group, Advisors and the NCEPOD Steering Group prior to publication.

The following grading system was used by the Advisors to grade the overall care each patient received.

**Good practice** – a standard that you would accept for yourself, your trainees and your institution
**Room for improvement** – aspects of clinical care that could have been better
**Room for improvement** – aspects of organisational care that could have been better
**Room for improvement** – aspects of both clinical and organisational care that could have been better
**Less than satisfactory** – several aspects of clinical and/or organisational care that were well below satisfactory

Insufficient information submitted to assess the quality of care.

## Quality and confidentiality

Each case was given a unique NCEPOD number so that cases could not easily be linked to a hospital.

The data from all questionnaires received were electronically scanned into a preset database. Prior to any analysis taking place, the data were cleaned to ensure that there were no duplicate records and that erroneous data had not been entered during scanning. Any fields in an individual record that contained spurious data that could not be validated were removed.

## Data analysis

The qualitative data collected from the Advisors' opinions and free text answers in the clinician questionnaires were coded, where applicable, according to content to allow quantitative analysis. The data were reviewed by NCEPOD Clinical Co-ordinators and a Clinical Researcher to identify the nature and frequency of recurring themes. Case studies have been used to illustrate particular themes.

## Data returns

Figure 1.1 shows the data returns for the study.

Over the three month period 5612 cases were reported of which 3404 were immediately excluded, usually because the patient had not undergone an appopriate procedure in the 30 days prior to death. A further 452 cases were found to be unsuitable and thus a total of 3856 patients were excluded. For included cases questionnaires were sent to the consultant surgeon and anaesthetist responsible for the patient's care and in total 63.7% of surgical and 60.8% of anaesthetic questionnaires were returned together with copied extracts of the case notes in 51.4% of cases; a complete data set was returned in only 600 cases.

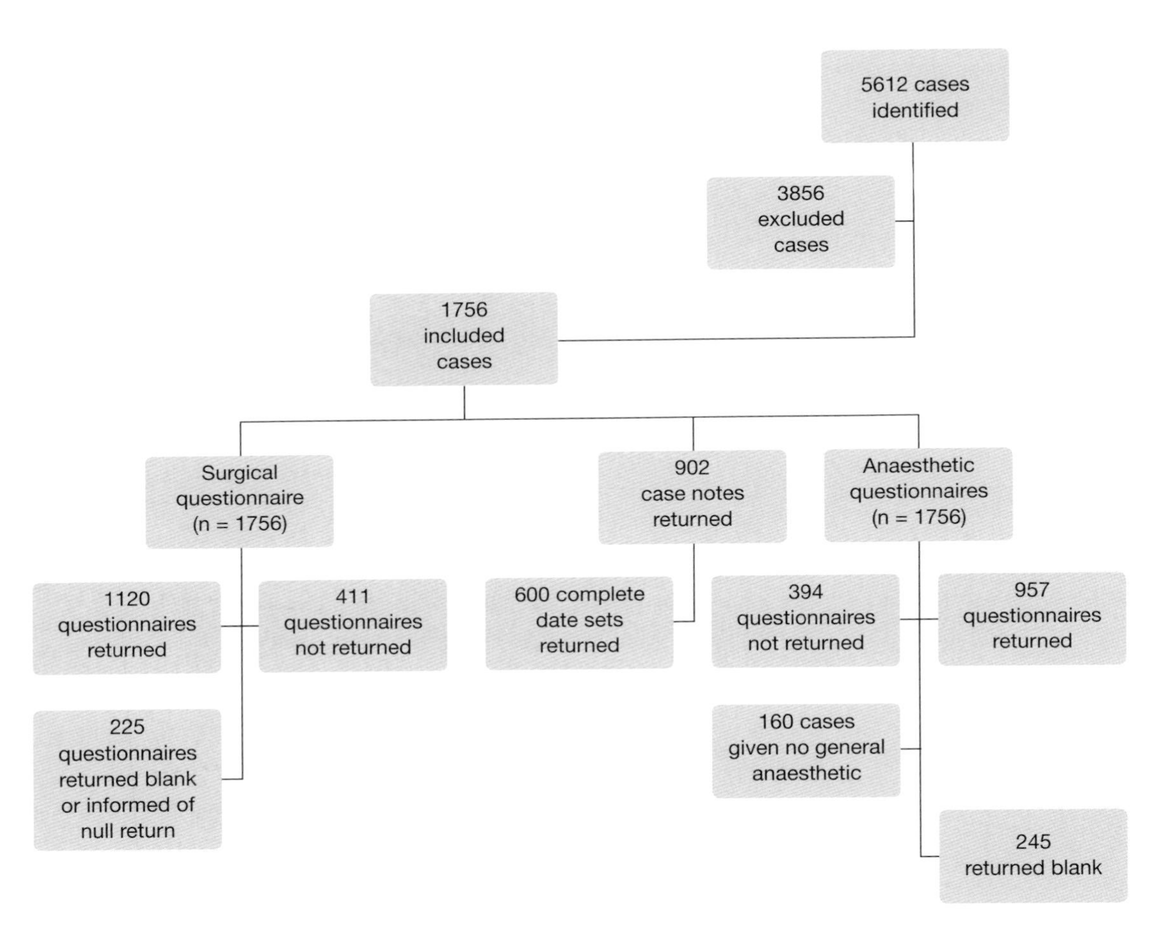


**Figure 1.1. Data returns**

In a number of cases questionnaires were returned blank to NCEPOD or we were informed of problems in terms of questionnaire completion; the most common reasons for this were case notes being lost or difficulty in retrieving case notes, and the consultant in charge of the patient at the time of their surgery no longer being at the hospital.

### Study sample denominator data by chapter

Within this report the denominator used in the analysis may change for each chapter and occasionally within each chapter. This is because data has been taken from different sources depending on the analysis required. For example in some cases the data presented will be a total from a question taken from the surgical or anaesthetic questionnaire only, whereas some analyses may have required a clinical questionnaire (either surgical or anaesthetic) and the Advisors' view taken from the case notes.

In total 820 cases were assessed by the Advisors. The remainder of the returned case note extracts (82 sets) were too incomplete for assessment. 1120 surgical questionnaires and 972 anaesthetic questionnaires were included in the analysis along with 283 organisational questionnaires.

## Study population and overall quality of care

### Age and gender

A majority (849/1120) of patients were aged between 80 – 89; 264/1120 patients were aged between 90 – 99; and 7 patients were aged over 100. 479/1120 of the sample was male and 641 female (Figure 1.2).

### Admission process

**Table 1.1 Urgency of admission**

| Urgency of admission | n | % |
|---|---|---|
| Elective | 157 | 14.0 |
| Planned | 27 | 2.4 |
| Emergency | 927 | 83.4 |
| **Subtotal** | **1111** | |
| Not answered | 9 | |
| **Total** | **1120** | |

The majority of the patients were admitted on an emergency basis (Table 1.1) via the emergency department or as a result of a direct referral from their

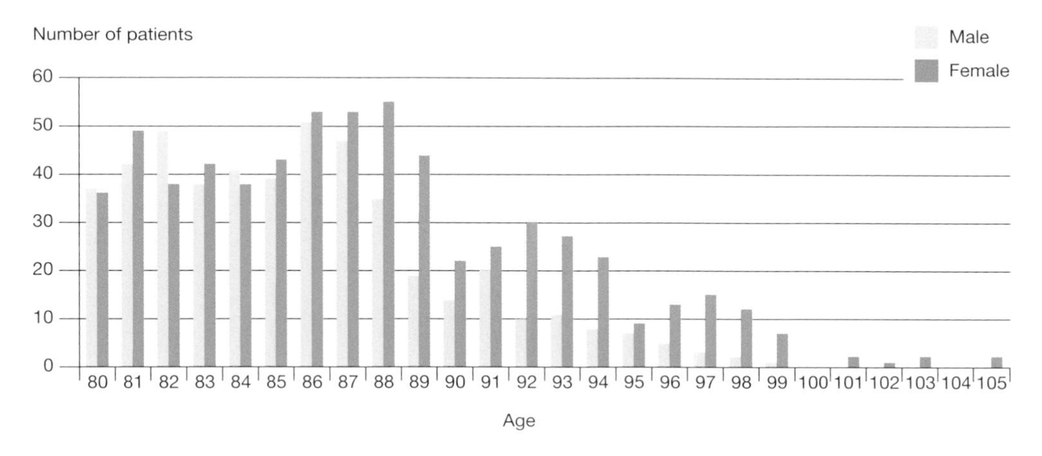


**Figure 1.2. Age and gender**

general medical or dental practitioner (Table 1.2). Surgeons were asked to assess the health status of the patient on admission using the American Society of Anaesthesiologists (ASA) score. A majority of patients (882/1085) were admitted with a severe systemic disease (ASA 3), or a severe systemic (ASA 4) disease that was a constant threat to life (Table 1.3).

**Table 1.2 Mode of admission**

| Mode of admission | n |
|---|---|
| Admission via the emergency department | 545 |
| Referral from general medical or dental practitioner | 200 |
| Admission following a previous outpatient consultation | 133 |
| Transfer as an inpatient from another hospital | 75 |
| Self referral by patient | 37 |
| Transferred from a nursing home | 36 |
| Readmission following inpatient stay | 27 |
| Planned readmission/routine follow up procedure | 14 |
| Tertiary (own specialty) | 8 |
| Unplanned admission following day case or outpatient procedure | 7 |
| Tertiary (other specialty) | 5 |
| Unplanned readmission following day case or outpatient procedure | 2 |
| Walk in clinic | 1 |
| Other | 25 |
| **Subtotal** | **1115** |
| Not answered | 5 |
| **Total** | **1120** |

**Table 1.3 Health status on admission**

| ASA on admission | n | % |
|---|---|---|
| ASA 1: a normal healthy patient | 4 | <1 |
| ASA 2: a patient with mild systemic disease | 170 | 15.7 |
| ASA 3: a patient with a severe systemic disease | 551 | 50.8 |
| ASA 4: a patient with a severe systemic disease that is a constant threat to life | 331 | 30.5 |
| ASA 5: a moribund patient who is not expected to survive the operation | 29 | 2.7 |
| **Subtotal** | **1085** | |
| Not answered | 35 | |
| **Total** | **1120** | |

## Operation undertaken

A breakdown of the most common operations undertaken is given in Table 1.4 which includes a group of patients who were considered to have undergone a more minor procedure.

**Table 1.4 Operation undertaken**

| Operation undertaken | n | % |
|---|---|---|
| Fractured neck of femur repair | 424 | 37.9 |
| Abdominal procedure | 349 | 31.2 |
| Other operation | 252 | 22.5 |
| Minor procedure | 95 | 8.5 |
| **Total** | **1120** | |

Throughout the report, the data presented on the whole group contains the subset of patients who underwent a minor procedure just as it does patients who underwent an operation for a fractured neck of femur or an acute abdomen. The data for minor procedures has been analysed separately to ensure these data were not skewing the overall picture and this was not found to be the case. The main differences were found around the expectation of survival (Table 1.5) and operative intent (Table 1.6).

**Table 1.5 Expectation of survival**

| Expected to survive | n | % |
|---|---|---|
| Yes | 33 | 37.5 |
| No | 17 | 19.3 |
| Unknown | 38 | 43.2 |
| **Subtotal** | **88** | |
| Not answered | 7 | |
| **Total** | **95** | |

There was a lower expectation of survival among those patients admitted for a more minor procedure than there was within the group as a whole; further to this operations were more likely to be carried out to help establish a diagnosis, and were much less likely to have a curative intent.

**Table 1.6 Operative intent**

| Operative intent | n | % |
|---|---|---|
| Diagnostic | 24 | 32.4 |
| Diagnostic and curative | 13 | 17.6 |
| Diagnostic and palliative | 3 | 4.1 |
| Curative | 19 | 25.7 |
| Palliative | 15 | 20.3 |
| **Subtotal** | **74** | |
| Not answered | 21 | |
| **Total** | **95** | |

## Number of days between operation and death

Just under 30% of the sample (220/740) died within the first three days of the procedure, and 52% (385/740) of the sample died within the first week of the operation (Figure 1.3).

## Overall assessment of care

As Figure 1.4 shows, only 37.5% (295/786) of the sample was assessed by Advisors as having received good care. 43.6% (343/786) of the sample was assessed as having room for improvement in either clinical or organisational care, and 12.5% (98/786) in aspects of both clinical and organisational care. 6.4% (50/786) of the sample was assessed by Advisors as having received care that was less than satisfactory. In 34 cases, the Advisors did not have enough information in the case notes to make an assessment of the overall level of care received.

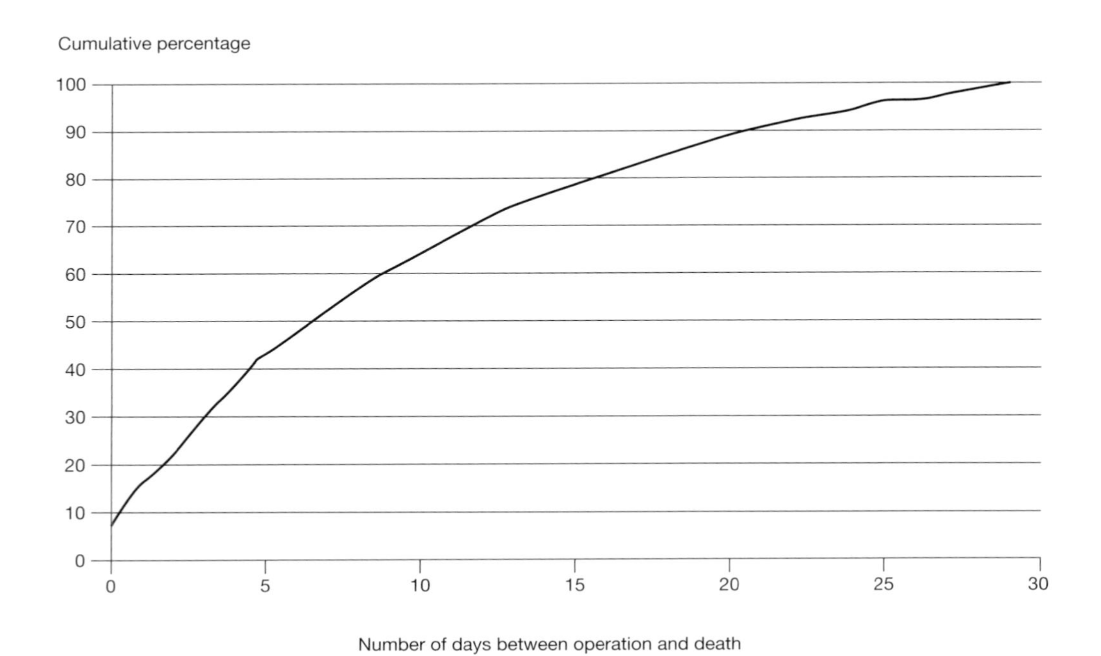


**Figure 1.3. Number of days between operation and death**

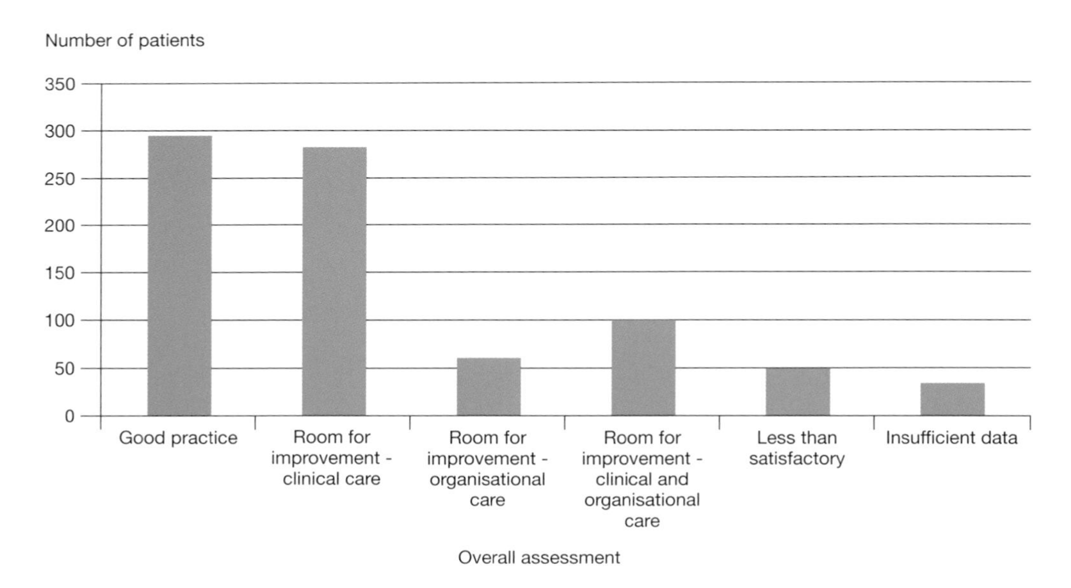


**Figure 1.4. Overall assessment of care**

# 2 – Hospital facilities & multidisciplinary care of the elderly

## Organisation of care for the elderly

365 sites participated in this study, (an additional 6 sites were participating at the beginning of the study, but closed during the course of the study). An organisational questionnaire was sent for completion to 361 sites (one Trust with four sites notified us of their participation too late to be sent organisational questionnaires); this questionnaire asked about the arrangements for care of surgical patients over 80 years of age. 283/361 (78.4%) were returned. Table 2.1 shows the number of returns by hospital type.

**Table 2.1 Organisational data returns by hospital type**

| Hospital type | n | % |
|---|---|---|
| District general (or equivalent) | 117 | 41.3 |
| University teaching hospital | 64 | 22.6 |
| Community | 7 | 2.5 |
| Limited surgical specialties | 20 | 7.1 |
| Independent | 68 | 24.0 |
| Other | 7 | 2.5 |
| **Total** | **283** | |

## Medicine for the Care of Older People (MCOP)

106/247 sites had no Medicine for the Care of Older People (MCOP) beds on the same site as surgery; (not answered by 36 sites). Of these, 75 reported that they had arrangements for review of pre- and post operative elderly patients and 16 sites had no such arrangements. In 5 sites it was unknown, and 10 sites did not answer this question.

Of those hospitals without MCOP on the same site that surgery was performed in elderly patients 49/106 were independent hospitals. However, 24 were District General Hospitals and 12 University Hospitals. The remaining 21 sites comprised 2 community hospitals, 16 sites offering limited surgical specialties and 3 sites which were classified as other.

101/261 sites stated that they had funded sessions for MCOP specifically to care for surgical patients (Table 2.2) and 143 did not.

**Table 2.2 Funded consultant sessions for MCOP care in surgical patients**

| Funded consultant sessions | n | % |
|---|---|---|
| Yes | 101 | 38.7 |
| No | 143 | 54.8 |
| Unknown | 17 | 6.5 |
| **Subtotal** | **261** | |
| Not answered | 22 | |
| **Total** | **283** | |

## Pre-operative assessment facilities

Of those sites that responded, only 2/225 sites had an upper age limit for admission to critical care, and 219 sites did not (in 4 sites this was unknown and 58 sites did not answer). Furthermore, 3/279 sites had a specific age limit above which day surgery was precluded regardless of comorbidities (274/279 had no age limit and this was not answered by 4 sites).

Of those sites that responded, 29/278 had a policy for medical pre-assessment in patients above a particular age (Table 2.3).

**Table 2.3 Existence of a policy for medical pre-assessment in patients above a certain age**

| Policy for medical pre-assessment | n | % |
|---|---|---|
| Yes | 29 | 10.4 |
| No | 243 | 87.4 |
| Unknown | 6 | 2.2 |
| **Subtotal** | **278** | |
| Not answered | 5 | |
| **Total** | **283** | |

The elderly patient undergoing surgery may have needs which are different to the general population; among these complex comorbidities, nutrition, comprehension and competence, and the avoidance of hypothermia are all particularly important.

Thirty sites did not have written policies or protocols for assessing the nutritional status of patients (Table 2.4), and 98/277 sites did not have a nutrition team (Table 2.5).

**Table 2.4 Existence of policies or protocols for assessing nutrition status**

| Policy for assessing nutritional status | n | % |
|---|---|---|
| Yes | 233 | 83.8 |
| No | 30 | 10.8 |
| Unknown | 15 | 5.4 |
| **Subtotal** | **278** | |
| Not answered | 5 | |
| **Total** | **283** | |

**Table 2.5 Presence of a nutrition team**

| Presence of a nutrition team | n | % |
|---|---|---|
| Yes | 174 | 62.8 |
| No | 98 | 35.4 |
| Unknown | 5 | 1.8 |
| **Subtotal** | **277** | |
| Not answered | 6 | |
| **Total** | **283** | |

A majority of hospitals had a policy for assessing the competence and comprehension of patients (Table 2.6); and of the 62/272 which did not, 21 were independent hospitals, 20 District General Hospitals, 13 University/ Teaching hospitals, 4 limited surgical specialties; 3 community and 1 other.

**Table 2.6 Policies for assessing the competence and comprehension of patients.**

| Policies for assessing competence and comprehension | n | % |
|---|---|---|
| Yes | 187 | 68.8 |
| No | 62 | 22.8 |
| Unknown | 23 | 8.5 |
| **Subtotal** | **272** | |
| Not answered | 11 | |
| **Total** | **283** | |

Nearly all sites (273/277) had clear guidelines in place for the assessment and consent of those patients with reduced capacity; this was unknown in 4 sites and not answered in 6.

Of the 250 sites where an answer was given, only 137 had a specific agreed integrated multidisciplinary care plan for patients with fractured neck of femur (fractured NOF) (Table 2.7).

**Table 2.7 Specific agreed integrated multidisciplinary care plans for patients with a fracture neck of femur**

| Multidisciplinary care pathway for fractured NOF | n | % |
|---|---|---|
| Yes | 137 | 54.8 |
| No | 106 | 42.4 |
| Unknown | 7 | 2.8 |
| **Subtotal** | **250** | |
| Not answered | 33 | |
| **Total** | **283** | |

Finally, less than two thirds (169/266) of sites had a cross directorate policy on the avoidance of peri-operative hypothermia (Table 2.8). Further comment is made on the topic of temperature monitoring and management in Chapter 5.

**Table 2.8 Presence of policies on the avoidance of peri-operative hypothermia**

| Policies on the avoidance of hypothermia | n | % |
|---|---|---|
| Yes | 169 | 63.5 |
| No | 73 | 27.4 |
| Unknown | 24 | 9.0 |
| **Subtotal** | **266** | |
| Not answered | 17 | |
| **Total** | **283** | |

## Post operative facilities

Planning for the safe discharge of the elderly patient is also vitally important.

The organisational questionnaire asked whether the hospital had access to beds in a geriatric orthopaedic rehabilitation unit or other intermediate care facility for the elderly.

**Table 2.9 Access to beds in a geriatric orthopaedic rehabilitation unit or other intermediate care facility for the elderly**

| Access to rehabilitation beds | n | % |
|---|---|---|
| Yes | 155 | 59.8 |
| No | 96 | 37.1 |
| Unknown | 8 | 3.1 |
| **Subtotal** | **259** | |
| Not answered | 24 | |
| **Total** | **283** | |

As Table 2.9 shows, 96 sites did not have access to any such beds.

Furthermore, although present in 216/275 sites, 47/275 sites did not have a policy for discharge planning in elderly patients; in 12 sites this was unknown and 8 sites did not answer this question.

## Multidisciplinary care of the elderly

The 2001 National Service Framework (NSF) for older people[1] recognised that care of the elderly in hospital is complex (standard 4). It recommended that older people be given the early supervision and advice of a specialist team when admitted to an acute general hospital. In particular it stated that there should be involvement of a consultant in old age medicine or rehabilitation, so that appropriate treatment and management decisions could be made. As well as medical consultants who care for the elderly, specialist nurses/nurse consultants; physiotherapists, occupational therapists and speech and language specialists; dieticians; social workers and care managers; and pharmacists are required. This provides a "comprehensive geriatric assessment" and has been shown to reduce hospital stay, readmission rates and long term institutionalisation. Further work in 2006 has emphasised the need to design services with the elderly in mind.[2]

Surgeons completing the questionnaire were asked if there was formal regular input from MCOP to the surgical care of patients. In 613/1076 this was the case, but in 395 it was not, and in 112 cases this was not answered or was unknown. We asked further what this constituted and allowed multiple answers. In 273 this included a weekly ward round, in 270 an on call referral service and in only 121 did MCOP have input into guidelines and policies. Despite the fact that all 3 types of service may have been available in some centres, the overall paucity of involvement, constituting no more than a weekly ward round or on call service for many, was noteworthy. Advisors were particularly concerned that so few units said that MCOP provided input into guidelines and policies. This suggested to us that systems of care did not benefit from multidisciplinary discussion, reflection and advance planning i.e. MCOP care was not properly embedded within surgical services.

Surgeons were also asked if patients who were not admitted under MCOP were reviewed by an MCOP consultant prior to surgery (Table 2.10).

**Table 2.10 Patient review by an MCOP physician**

| Reviewed by an MCOP physician | n | % |
|---|---|---|
| Yes | 225 | 23.3 |
| No | 653 | 67.7 |
| Unknown | 87 | 9.0 |
| **Subtotal** | **965** | |
| Not answered | 121 | |
| **Total** | **1086** | |

In 225/1086 the patient was reviewed by MCOP, in 653 they were not, and in 87 cases this was unknown (34 patients were admitted under the care of MCOP). Advisors were asked if they found evidence of the involvement of MCOP clinicians in their review of case notes. This was found in only 138/774 cases pre-operatively and 212/744 cases post- operatively; Advisors were unable to answer or did not answer the question in a further 76 cases. This suggested that MCOP involvement often only occurred when problems arose post operatively, and/or that the documentation of involvement was poor.

The recent incorporation of the care standards into Best Practice Tariff for the care of fractured neck of femur by the Department of Heath in England[3] is welcomed (April 2010).[2,4]

To ensure full tariff the following domains need to be included within the care pathway for fractured femur in the elderly:

- Admitted under the joint care of a Consultant Geriatrician and a Consultant Orthopaedic Surgeon
- Admitted using an assessment protocol agreed by geriatric medicine, orthopaedic surgery and anaesthesia
- Assessed by a Geriatrician in the peri-operative period - Geriatrician defined as consultant, non consultant career grade, or ST3+; Peri-operative period defined as within 72 hours of admission
- Post operative Geriatrician-directed: Multiprofessional rehabilitation team and Fracture prevention assessments (falls and bone health)

The involvement of MCOP clinicians for particular diagnostic groups was examined. Overall surgeons reported that MCOP had some input in 613/1076 patients (Table 2.11). In those patients where the diagnosis was fractured neck of femur (n=424) involvement was more likely to be available (351/420 cases; not answered in 4 cases) than in general surgical patients undergoing emergency surgery for an acute abdomen (n=274) (81/265 cases, not answered in 9 cases).

**Table 2.11 Formal regular input from MCOP to the surgical team**

| Formal MCOP input | n | % |
|---|---|---|
| Yes | 613 | 57.0 |
| No | 395 | 36.7 |
| Unknown | 68 | 6.3 |
| **Subtotal** | **1076** | |
| Not answered | 44 | |
| **Total** | **1120** | |

In the opinion of Advisors specialist teams should have been involved in the care of the patient in 232/750 cases (no in 518 cases, unable to answer or not answered in 70 cases in which it did not occur). Most Advisors suggested that further involvement by MCOP/General Medicine (specialties) would have been beneficial (131), with a minority suggesting palliative care (14), critical care (10) surgical specialties (9) and anaesthesia (7). In 77 cases the Advisors did not note the particular team that should have been involved.

A recent model of care has demonstrated the ability of high quality multidisciplinary input to improve the peri-operative care of elderly patients undergoing elective orthopaedic surgery.[5] As well as reducing length of stay, there was a reduction in delirium, post operative pneumonia and pressure sores in the group receiving the enhanced programme. Pain control was also improved, urinary catheter use reduced and mobilisation occurred earlier. It is particularly laudable that this was successful in the context of a very large teaching hospital.

## Key findings

There was a relative paucity of MCOP involvement within this sample of patients at all stages of care despite the recommendations included in the NSF for the Elderly.

Mechanisms for the assessment of nutrition and mental capacity were absent in a number of sites, (30/278 and 62/272 respectively).

## Recommendations

Routine daily input from Medicine for the Care of Older People should be available to elderly patients undergoing surgery and is integral to inpatient care pathways in this population. (Trusts and Clinical Directors)

All hospitals should address the need for nutrition and mental capacity to be assessed and documented in the elderly on admission as a minimum standard. (Trusts and Clinical Directors)

### *References*


1. Department of Health. *The National Service Framework for older people*. 2001. Crown Copyright.

2. The Department of Health. *A new ambition for old age: Next steps in implementing the National Service Framework for older people*. 2006. Crown Copyright.

3. Best Practice Tariff (BPT) for Fragility Hip Fracture Care. Department of Health 2010. http://webarchive.nationalarchives.gov.uk/+/www.dh.gov.uk/en/Managingyourorganisation/Financeandplanning/NHSFinancialReforms/DH_105080

4. Scottish Intercollegiate Guidelines Network. *Management of hip fracture in older people. A national clinical guideline. 2009. Scottish Intercollegiate Guidelines Network*

5. Harari D, Hopper A, Dhesi J, Babic-Illman G, Lockwood L & Martin F. Proactive care of older people undergoing surgery ('POPS'): Designing, embedding, evaluating and funding a comprehensive geriatric assessment service for older elective surgical patients. *Age and Ageing*, 2007; 36(2), 190 - 196

# 3 – Patient comorbidities

When elderly patients present for surgery many have other significant comorbidities. It has been estimated that by the age of 75 years >50% of the population have a limiting longstanding illness.[1] It is generally believed that cardio-respiratory disease has most relevance to the incidence of serious post operative complications and adverse outcomes, and that these patients require particularly careful preoperative assessment.[2,3] However other common health considerations include diabetes, dementia, sensory impairment, mental health problems, incontinence, stroke and arthritis.[4,5,6,7,8] These latter problems often result in disabilities or functional impairment which complicate recovery and make outcome less predictable. The weight of comorbidity and disability together with the limitation of activities co-incident with loss of physiological reserve needs to be fully explored and taken into account in the peri-operative care of the elderly.

## Physiological reserve

The normal effects of ageing result in important changes in functional reserve.[9] These may be thought of as a reduction in the gap between basal and maximal organ performance. Even the fit elderly patient is less able to adjust cardiac output in relation to fluid shifts and infection, and more prone to cardiac ischaemia and arrhythmias. The "well" elderly patient is also more prone to hypoxia and pulmonary infection, and other vital organ dysfunction after major surgery. Patients are more likely to suffer the effects of mild and reversible renal and cognitive impairment, and these in turn may be compounded by the effects of multiple medications, which behave differently as a result of the pharmacokinetic and dynamic changes consequent upon increasing age.

## Frailty

Frailty is common with advanced age and in a western population it has been estimated that 10-15% of the over 80's are frail, with around 1% - 4.4% very frail.[10] It presents an increasingly well recognised pattern of nutritional, medical and functional problems.[11] At all ages women are at an increased risk. Although a widely used term, definitions may appear relatively broad and non specific. Scoring systems incorporate risk factors for frailty e.g. low and high body mass, poor muscle strength, memory loss, loss of cognition, and anaemia. These factors as well as the "end of bed" assessment of frailty have been linked to outcomes including increased risk of death, falls and institutionalisation.[12,13]

Whilst it is important to identify frailty as an entity, we note that it is variously defined; for example by operational means (Figure 3.1[14]), frailty scales (which are generally complex and summate up to 70 parameters (e.g. the "Frailty index[15]) and clinical judgement.

---

Frailty exists when the patient displays any 3 of the following:

- Unintentional weight loss (at least 4kg in last year)
- Self reported exhaustion
- Weak grip strength
- Slow walking speed
- Low physical activity[14]

**Figure 3.1. The Canadian Veterans Heart Study Definition of frailty**

---

In the Canadian study of age and ageing[15] each category of frailty increases the risk of death or institutionalisation by 20% within a 6 year time frame. This scale (which was not developed within a surgical population) has been shown to perform better than (single) measures of cognition, function or comorbidity in assessing risk of death.

Surgeons completing the questionnaire were asked as part of their overall assessment of the patient whether they had identified frailty on admission. A large number of those patients in which a surgical questionnaire was returned (703/1063) were noted to be frail (Table 3.1).

The most common method of assessing frailty was by history and examination, and specific scoring systems were not cited.

Advisors were asked whether they considered from examination of records, there had been clear recognition of risk factors for frailty in patients (Table 3.2).

In large numbers of patients these risk factors were identified; in 304/536 records the Advisors considered there to be clear recognition by the admitting team of poor nutrition; in 478/600 cases there was thought to be poor mobility, and in 391/523 there was clear recognition by the admitting team of memory loss or dementia.

**Table 3.1 Patient identified as being frail**

| Frailty identified | n | % |
|---|---|---|
| Yes | 703 | 66.1 |
| No | 195 | 18.3 |
| Unknown | 165 | 15.5 |
| **Subtotal** | **1063** | |
| Not answered | 57 | |
| **Total** | **1120** | |

Whilst frailty was recognised, it may not have been sufficiently factored into risk assessments, and subsequent optimal planning of care. An overall assessment of frailty has been strongly linked to outcomes which are relevant in both surgical and non surgical settings. Although frailty is a risk factor for disability, there may not be an absolute association between frailty, comorbidity and disability. Frailty should be more clearly understood as an independent and additional risk factor for poor outcome.[16,17]

**Table 3.2 Advisors' opinion on clear recognition by the admitting team of risk factors for frailty in the patient**

| Clear recognition | Poor nutritional status | | Immobility | | Memory loss or dementia | |
|---|---|---|---|---|---|---|
| | n | % | n | % | n | % |
| Yes | 304 | 56.7 | 478 | 79.7 | 391 | 74.8 |
| No | 232 | 43.3 | 122 | 20.3 | 132 | 25.2 |
| **Subtotal** | **536** | | **600** | | **523** | |
| Unable to answer | 244 | | 181 | | 240 | |
| Not answered | 40 | | 39 | | 57 | |
| **Total** | **820** | | **820** | | **820** | |

The following case study describes a patient who was noted to be "frail". Whilst this was mentioned in the admission notes it was clear to Advisors that peri-operative planning had not considered how outcome from major surgery might be optimised for the patient taking this into account.

**Case study 1**

A patient was admitted semi-electively for right hemicolectomy for advanced cancer of the colon having had a colonic stent for obstruction 10 weeks previously. The patient was known to have liver metastases, had lost a considerable amount of weight and weighed 36kg. The patient was described as "frail" by the anaesthetist pre-operatively. After undergoing a 3.5 hour procedure which involved resection of the spleen due to adherent tumour the patient returned to the ward for "routine post op care". 24 hours post operatively the patient became oxygen dependent and developed surgical emphysema. A chest X ray revealed a left sided pleural effusion. On the 4th post operative day an anastomotic leak was recognised and on day 5 ICU care TPN was considered. On day 6 active treatment was withdrawn.

*Whilst having little in the way of specific (medical) comorbidity this patient was clearly grossly undernourished, and the anaesthetist commented on the overall "frailty" at pre-assessment. Why then were appropriate measures not taken to improve the chance of survival when undertaking such major surgery?*

# Specific comorbidity

## Anaemia

It is uncertain whether anaemia is a marker or a mediator of disease, but it is known to be relatively common in the elderly community with an incidence of approximately 17% in females and 28% in males according to World Health Organisation (WHO) definitions[18] (Haemoglobin (Hb) of <13 for females and <14 for males). More recently authors have linked anaemia with poorer outcome in old age, and particularly in males.[19] Anaemia is also often included as a risk factor within the assessment of general frailty in the elderly, alongside other risk factors such as low body mass and reduced strength/mobility. In a non surgical context it has been associated with an increased chance of serious events in elderly patients with cardiac disease (in particular heart failure and angina) and in the operative setting, even relatively minor degrees of anaemia have been associated with increased mortality in patients having major non cardiac surgery.[20] In the current study population the percentage of patients with a haemoglobin concentration less than 12g/dl was 54%, (520/957) with 17% (163/957) less than 10g/dl and in 3.1% (30/957) less than 8g/dl.

Whilst pre-operative anaemia is more common in the elderly there has generally been a more conservative approach to the risks and benefits of blood transfusion in all patients in the last 10-15 years, and in an intensive care setting transfusion triggers of around 9 g/dl have been commonly applied to patients irrespective of age.[21] Based on physiological decline (in particular reduced cardiac and pulmonary reserve) as well as additional specific comorbidity, there may be a need to set a higher transfusion trigger in the elderly. This is a complex area, and current literature is unclear. We feel that additional review specific to the elderly is required, and that there are reasons to be cautious in applying unrealistically low transfusion triggers in this population.

**Case study 2**

A patient with a past history of angina, heart failure and chronic obstructive pulmonary disease presented with a fractured neck of femur. The pre-operative haemoglobin was 12.5 g/dl. The patient underwent surgery in a timely fashion under general anaesthesia and regional blockade but developed atrial fibrillation 3 days post operatively and became acutely breathless with a diagnosis of acute heart failure. Haemoglobin at this stage was noted to be 7.5g/dl and clinical signs of a cerebrovascular accident (CVA) developed 5 days post operatively. Further active treatment was discontinued.

Whilst it would have been extremely unusual to have needed to transfuse this patient in the peri-operative period, their relative anaemia in the presence of cardiopulmonary disease may have contributed to their demise.

*Advisors commented that they would have expected that both haemoglobin and electrolytes should be routinely checked in patients at least once in the first 24 hours post operatively.*

*There are many reasons why this patient with complex medical problems sustained a CVA post operatively. However Advisors commented that the patient's low haemoglobin may have contributed to the poor outcome and that it should have been both noted and actively managed.*

## Other comorbidities

1028/1098 patients had at least one comorbidity at the time of admission (44 no comorbidities, 26 unknown and in 22 cases unanswered). The most common comorbidities are identified in Table 3.3.

Percentages were calculated for 1001/1028 patients where there was comorbidity and the clinician completing the questionnaire indicated what this was. The incidence of cardiopulmonary and cerebrovascular disease was particularly high in this population, and the fact that many comorbidities co-existed emphasise the complexity of the problems faced by the clinicians caring for them, and their increased peri-operative risk.[22] Most of these patients would also have been receiving specific drug treatments which further complicate their management.

Of particular note is the incidence of renal impairment (22%) which will be specifically discussed with fluid balance in Chapters 4 and 6. Renal disease was not explicitly defined in our questionnaire, but was based on a raised serum creatinine and/or a marked reduction in urine output.

In the 1999 Extremes of Age report, in a population of patients over 90 years, categorisation of comorbidity was less detailed but it was reported that 57% had cardiac, 28% respiratory and 18% neurological problems. 12% had renal impairment, and 13% "psychiatric" disease.[23]

Table 3.3 Comorbidities present at the time of admission

| Comorbidity | n* | % |
|---|---|---|
| Ischaemic Heart Disease | 814 | 81.3 |
| Hypertension | 478 | 47.8 |
| Respiratory disease | 280 | 28.0 |
| Renal disease | 217 | 21.7 |
| Previous Transient Ischaemic Attack (TIA) & Stroke | 197 | 19.7 |
| Dementia | 185 | 18.5 |
| Memory impairment | 144 | 14.4 |
| Diabetes | 136 | 13.6 |
| Osteoporosis or previous bone fracture | 132 | 13.2 |
| Parkinson's disease | 24 | 2.4 |
| Delirium | 23 | 2.3 |
| Not answered | 27 | |

**answers may be multiple*

### Disability

Many patients over 80 also have specific disabilities and the prevalence increases with age. In part as a result of these disabilities, the elderly patient may have a very much reduced ability to retain their autonomy after illness, and many cannot return to the same functional level. Early recognition is important to facilitate immediate care and for discharge planning and rehabilitation.[24] However the documentation of disabilities may be poor, particularly if the patient is acutely unwell.

### Daily living

Advisors found evidence of difficulties in basic functions of daily living prior to admission in 43% (322/733) of this population. There was no evidence of any difficulty in 411 cases, unable to answer in 80 and did not answer in 7.

Sensory impairment such as hearing and visual loss are increasingly prevalent with age and contribute significantly to other physical disabilities, as well as complicating communication. Hearing loss (the most common sensory impairment in the elderly) and/or visual loss occurs in many elderly patients. Hearing loss is present as many as 50-75% of the over 80s and bilateral visual loss may occur in up to 30% of patients over 65.[25,26] However recognition may be a problem, particularly of hearing loss where there is a relatively low use of hearing aids. Visual loss may be secondary to cataracts and presbyopia, glaucoma, diabetic eye disease and age related macular degeneration.

**Table 3.4 Advisors' opinion on evidence of sensory impairment**

| Sensory impairment | | Visual impairment (n) | | | | | |
|---|---|---|---|---|---|---|---|
| | | Yes | No | Subtotal | Unable to answer | Not answered | Total |
| Hearing impairment (n) | Yes | 33 | 67 | 100 | 9 | 13 | 122 |
| | No | 42 | 6 | 48 | 0 | 0 | 48 |
| | Subtotal | 75 | 73 | 148 | 9 | 13 | 170 |
| | Unable to answer | 3 | 0 | 3 | 6 | 0 | 9 |
| | Not answered | 10 | 0 | 10 | 0 | 2 | 12 |
| | Total | 88 | 73 | 161 | 15 | 15 | 191 |

In the current study Advisors assessing the cases found documented evidence of some form of sensory loss in 191/718 patients; in 101 they were unable to answer and in one case did not answer the question. Of the 191,122/170 had hearing loss, and 88/161 had visual loss; 33/148 patients had evidence of both hearing and visual loss (Table 3.4). This was almost certainly an underestimate. Documentation of disabilities is also likely to have been poor in the medical notes particularly in the context of acute illness. Nevertheless hearing and visual loss constitute significant ongoing problems and affect both immediate day to day care and recovery. They should be both sought and documented and clearly communicated to the hospital team.

As well as hearing and visual loss elderly patients may suffer additional problems such as dysarthria secondary to stroke and Parkinson's disease which may further complicate communication.

Other communication problems were documented in nearly a quarter of our population (Table 3.5). It is self evident that patients with these problems require skilled assistance when hospitalised.

**Table 3.5 Advisors' opinion on other sensory potential communication or perception problems**

| Other communication or perception problems | n | % |
|---|---|---|
| Yes | 175 | 23.7 |
| No | 562 | 76.3 |
| **Subtotal** | **737** | |
| Unable to answer | 68 | |
| Not answered | 15 | |
| **Total** | **820** | |

## Dementia and memory impairment

The prevalence of dementia is estimated at about 11% in those aged 80-84 and as high as 24% in the over 85 age group. Currently there are approximately 700,000 individuals with dementia in the UK and this is set to increase to 1.4 million by 2040.[27,28,29]

A number of patients in this study were noted to have dementia or memory loss complicating their surgical care. At the time of admission dementia was noted in 185/1001 and memory impairment in 144/1001 patients; including 23 patients who had both dementia and memory impairment. A total of 323/1001 patients had some form of cognitive impairment, (Table 3.3).

Admission to hospital may precipitate confusion and even delirium in some elderly patients and those with pre-existing dementia or memory loss are at most risk. Delirium is best managed by the avoidance of sedative drugs and if at all possible medical interventions (such as urinary catheterisation).[30,31]

If confusion or delirium were present pre-operatively Advisors were asked if based on the information available in the case notes, this was well managed. In 85/179 patients this was confirmed by Advisors to be the case (Table 3.6).

**Table 3.6 Advisors' opinion on the management of confusion or delirium**

| Well managed | n | % |
|---|---|---|
| Yes | 85 | 47.5 |
| No | 94 | 52.5 |
| **Subtotal** | **179** | |
| Unable to answer | 156 | |
| Not answered | 111 | |
| Not applicable | 374 | |
| **Total** | **820** | |

Case study 3 illustrates a typical patient with risk factors for delirium.

**Case study 3**

A non English speaking patient was admitted under the care of MCOP with a history of recent immobility and confusion. Communication was difficult as there was no interpreter. A normal Glasgow Coma Score was noted, but the patient had a poor test of mental function (though this was difficult to be sure of due to language difficulties). After 5 days a diagnosis of septic arthritis of the knee was made and an arthroscopic washout was undertaken within 24 hours. Post operatively the patient was more confused, developed acute kidney injury 2 days post operatively and conscious level fluctuated. The diagnosis of multi organ failure secondary to sepsis was diagnosed. An end of life care pathway was commenced 7 days post operatively after discussion with the patient's family.

*Advisors commented on the lack of involvement of senior clinicians in this case, and the paucity of basic skills in the trainees caring for the patient.*

## Post Operative Cognitive Dysfunction (POCD)

Confusion is likely to be more common after surgery and anaesthesia and has been noted in as many as 25% of patients.[32,33] It is more common in patients with a history of cognitive impairment, in those aged over 75, and patients having a second procedure or undergoing a lengthy anaesthetic.[34,35] It is also much more common in those with pre-operative confusion, and frailty. Recent research has cast doubt as to whether there is a difference between regional and general anaesthesia in the incidence of POCD.[35,36,37,38]

Evidence of post operative delirium and confusion was present in at least 287/909 patients in this study (Table 3.7).

**Table 3.7 Evidence of delirium or confusion**

| Evidence of delirium or confusion | n | % |
|---|---|---|
| Yes | 287 | 31.6 |
| No | 497 | 54.7 |
| Unknown | 125 | 13.8 |
| **Subtotal** | **909** | |
| Not answered | 211 | |
| **Total** | **1120** | |

## Cognition

In elderly patients, assessment and documentation of mental impairment on admission may be useful. This can be used to provide a baseline, and to assist with future communication. Advisors were asked if there was evidence that such an assessment was made. Whilst this was carried out in 395/701, there was no evidence that it was performed in a further 306 cases (Table 3.8).

**Table 3.8 Advisors' opinion on whether an assessment of mental capacity/impairment was made on admission**

| Assessment of mental capacity | n | % |
|---|---|---|
| Yes | 395 | 56.3 |
| No | 306 | 43.7 |
| **Subtotal** | **701** | |
| Unable to answer | 119 | |
| **Total** | **820** | |

It has been noted already that 323/1001 patients had dementia and/or memory loss documented on admission (Table 3.3). Others had sensory and or motor problems which would have produced significant communication problems. Signs may be subtle and such information may or may not be handed over clearly by those who have been caring for the patient prior to admission. Therefore an assessment and documentation of cognition and particular difficulties with communication is essential in all patients on admission, but particularly so in the elderly surgical population in whom we have already noted a high incidence of peri-operative confusion.

## Consent

Cognition is important within any assessment of capacity, which in turn is very important during the consent process.

It is also important to distinguish between lack of capacity and difficulty with communication. Where appropriate, specialists should assist in making an assessment of capacity (for example when doubt exists), and unless the urgency of the situation prevents it, the patient should be assisted to make and communicate their own decision wherever possible.[39]

If it has been decided that a patient lacks capacity then treatment decisions should be made in the patients best interests. "Best interests" extends beyond consideration of likely benefits and burdens of treatment and should also include consideration of the patient's wishes (past and present) and if known, any beliefs they may have which would have been likely to influence the decision. Treatment provided under these circumstances should be no more than is proportionate and necessary to the circumstances. When there is a lack of consensus about what is in the patient's best interests, or where serious decisions are being made about treatment and the patient has no one to speak for them, there may be a need to seek advice from an Independent Mental Capacity advocate. However this is not necessary when emergency treatment is required, when the standard common law duty to act in the patient's best interests applies. Within this study we reviewed cases where there was doubt about whether the patient's own wishes and "best interest" were indeed properly served. Case study 4 presents such an example.

**Case study 4**

A patient presented with vomiting and a strangulated femoral hernia. There was concern that there was a disseminated malignancy which involved the lumbar and thoracic spine. Surgery was initially declined by the patient but nevertheless went ahead 24 hours later under local anaesthesia, by which time the patient's conscious level had deteriorated, and the patient's ability to consent was reduced. At operation ischaemic bowel was discovered and treatment (latterly) discontinued.

*The fact that the patient "only had it under local" may have persuaded staff that this was an ethical decision, but Advisors believed that there was insufficient documentation to judge whether the patient's original wishes had been re-considered prior to surgery proceeding.*

In practice should the patient lack capacity and require urgent treatment, as much information as possible should be sought from relatives and carers about the wishes of the patient e.g. it should be known whether an advance directive is in place. Assuming that the treatment proposed is in the best interest of the patient, it should be discussed with members of the secondary care team, and when appropriate with carers and relatives. If no advance directive is in place, medical staff should then complete the consent form on behalf of the patient.

In this study we asked surgeons whether cognitive function was assessed at the point of consent. This was noted as having occurred in only 578/1046 cases. It was not assessed in a further 261 cases and it was unknown in 207 cases. Surgeons completing the questionnaire did not answer this question in 77 cases. It is probable that this assessment was more likely to have been formally undertaken in those with obvious or reported memory loss or dementia. Nevertheless, and particularly with regard to the age of this population, this is a relatively low number of cases.

Where cognitive function was assessed, further detail as to how this was carried out was collected and in the vast majority of cases this was by clinical assessment with or without a score such as the "Mini Mental Assessment" (Table 3.9).

**Table 3.9 Assessment of the patient's cognitive function**

| Type of assessment | n* |
|---|---|
| Clinical assessment | 432 |
| Mini Mental score | 158 |
| Other | 38 |

*answers may be multiple*

A clear (written) statement on cognitive ability and capacity and how it was assessed is extremely helpful for all those subsequently caring for patients, and ought to be presented as a matter of routine. However it should be stressed that capacity may vary in time both in relation to the patient and also the level of decision required where the same level of understanding may not be applicable to all decisions. Use of simple scoring systems can be useful in identifying less obvious problems with cognition but may not detect subtle memory loss, and are less good within certain educational and cultural groups. For example well educated individuals may score relatively well despite memory loss. The Mental Capacity Act[40] provides guidance and states that a patient will be capable to decide if they:

- Can understand the information relevant to the decision
- Can retain this information even if for only a short space of time
- Can use or weigh the information relevant to the decision making process including seeing both sides of the argument and being able to make a decision one way or the other
- Can communicate their decision by talking or other means of communication e.g. sign language

As well as asking whether cognitive function was assessed on admission, the surgeon completing the questionnaire was also asked whether patients had been assessed as competent to consent to surgery. Whilst just 578 patients had had cognitive function assessed at the time of consent, 756 were ultimately deemed able to consent (Table 3.10).

**Table 3.10 Judgement on whether the patient was competent to consent to surgery**

| Patient judged competent to consent | n | % |
|---|---|---|
| Yes | 756 | 72.1 |
| No | 249 | 23.7 |
| Unknown | 44 | 4.2 |
| **Subtotal** | **1049** | |
| Not answered | 71 | |
| **Total** | **1120** | |

Systems employed to take consent were examined in more detail in the 249 cases where the patient had been deemed incompetent (Table 3.11). In the majority of cases the correct process was followed and a second doctor signed the consent in the best interests of the patient. However, there were 28 cases where the next of kin consented and 10 cases where a relative or carer was asked to consent. Relatives should not be asked to sign a consent form on behalf of an adult who lacks capacity to consent themselves unless they have been given authority to do so under a Lasting Power of Attorney or as a "Court appointed deputy". Nevertheless good practice generally includes full discussion with family members as to what surgery is proposed, what the patient's wishes might have been, and possible outcomes.

**Table 3.11 Person giving signed consent if the patient lacked capacity**

| Person giving consent | n* |
|---|---|
| Surgeon in the best interest of the patient | 192 |
| Another medical colleague | 30 |
| Next of kin | 28 |
| Family or carers | 10 |
| Other | 3 |

**answers may be multiple*

Revised guidance on the consent process was published in England and Wales in 2001[41], and further advice was issued in June 2009[42] in line with additional legislation including the Mental Capacity Act which became law in October 2007.[40] Specific advice also exists on the particular needs within the consent process in the elderly,[43] but this should be referred to in association with the 2009 guidance.

Data for this study was collected just 1 year after the Mental Capacity Act came into force, but prior to the revised DH consent guidance. In line with this guidance it is suggested that the documentation of competence which underpins the consent process ought to be much more explicit, stating both the method of assessment used (which should be standardised) and the result.

There was very little evidence of the use of advance directives or living wills. Only 20/1077 patients included in this study were noted to have one. It was unknown whether one was present in 550 cases, and not answered in 43 cases.

## Prescribing in the elderly

As expected, given the level of comorbidity in this population, some patients were on relatively large numbers of medicines pre-operatively. Based on assessment of the hospital drug charts, 463/740 patients were prescribed > 5 drugs (The NSF for the elderly suggests that >4 is "polypharmacy"[44]). This may not be surprising given the need for additional medication such as anticoagulants, analgesics, and oxygen in the pre-operative period. However 149 patients were on more than 10 medications (Table 3.12). This highlights the very real possibility of medicine errors and serious interactions.[45] It also points to the burden of care for these patients, where much nursing time may be spent administering medications in any 24 hour period.

**Table 3.12 How many medications was the patient prescribed pre-operatively? – Advisors' opinion**

| Number of medications prescribed pre-operatively | n | % |
|---|---|---|
| 1- 5 | 277 | 37.4 |
| >5 | 314 | 42.4 |
| >10 | 149 | 20.1 |
| **Subtotal** | **740** | |
| Unable to answer | 79 | |
| Not answered | 1 | |
| **Total** | **820** | |

The reasons for polypharmacy are multi-factorial but include chronic diseases requiring particular treatments, more than one physician involved in medical care (a particular problem in the peri-operative period), failure to review medication and discontinue unnecessary drugs, and adherence to evidence based medicine without clear thought about the burden to the patient and the potential for side effects and interaction. This may result in what has been termed a "prescribing cascade".[46,47] Senior and regular examination of prescribing is required and should include a review of the patient, noting the risks as well as benefits. Our Advisors also strongly endorsed the input of an experienced ward pharmacist.

**Case study 5**

A patient with an ischaemic leg was admitted to a surgical ward for amputation, with a history of cardiac failure, chronic renal impairment (creatinine 185 micromoles/L), Parkinsons disease and temporal arteritis, and was receiving 14 medications on admission (excluding analgesics).

Risk factors for AKI were recognised but this did not prevent it's development post operatively.

*Advisors commented that the complexity of this patient's condition, coupled with the large number of prescribed medications required earlier senior review by clinicians with the relevent expertise.*

Although questions relating to weight were not asked in relation to drug dosage it was found that weight was often not recorded (Chapter 4, Table 4.18). Body weight is an essential basic measurement on which many fluid and drug dose calculations are made in the peri-operative period. In particular the elderly patient is often underweight, and whilst absolute measurements may be difficult in the sick immobile patient estimates can be made. Those admitted from care facilities should have had weight recorded regularly prior to admission.[48] For the immobile hospitalised patient bed scales should also be more widely available, and would also assist with fluid balance peri-operatively.

With respect to post operative drugs it was of note that a relatively large proportion of patients were prescribed post operative oxygen therapy 725/879 (Table 3.13). Post operative oxygen therapy when administered after major surgery may reduce peri-operative cardiorespiratory morbidity. This effect may be particularly beneficial in the elderly who are already "physiologically challenged".

**Table 3.13 Prescription of post operative oxygen therapy**

| Prescribed post operative oxygen therapy | n | % |
|---|---|---|
| Yes | 725 | 82.5 |
| No | 117 | 13.3 |
| Unknown | 37 | 4.2 |
| **Subtotal** | **879** | |
| Not answered | 78 | |
| **Total** | **957** | |

Pre and post operative oxygen therapy has also been shown to reduce POCD.[49]

A number of patients (150/862) were prescribed post operative sedatives including benzodiazepines (Table 3.14). These may have been used to treat post operative agitation and confusion but may have also contributed to the problem.[50] Some may also have been prescribed before admission to hospital and prescriptions continued without further consideration. Effects are unpredictable and may be cumulative when sedative agents are used alongside other centrally acting drugs such as antidepressants, anticholinergics, antipsychotics and opioids.

**Table 3.14 Benzodiazepines or any sedatives other than opiates administered post operatively**

| Post operative sedatives administered | n | % |
|---|---|---|
| Yes | 150 | 17.4 |
| No | 683 | 79.2 |
| Unknown | 29 | 3.4 |
| **Subtotal** | **862** | |
| Not answered | 95 | |
| **Total** | **957** | |

## Key findings

Comorbidity was extremely common in the elderly surgical population included in this study (1028/1098).

"Frailty" was clearly and independently identified in our study population

Disabilities (Including hearing and visual loss) were common, not well documented and may have led to difficulties in caring for the elderly in the peri-operative period within this group of patients.

Acute illness in the elderly was complicated by pre-existing memory loss and dementia, both of which predispose to confusion in the peri-operative period. In this sample, 185/1001 and 144/1001 were documented as having dementia and/or memory loss.

Documentation of mental capacity in this sample was poor (395/701). When patients were unable to consent independently the correct procedures were followed in the majority of cases.

Some patients in this study were receiving a large variety of medicines (463/740), with a serious risk of drug interactions.

## Recommendations

Comorbidity, disability and frailty need to be clearly recognised and seen as independent markers of risk in the elderly. This requires skill and multidisciplinary input including early involvement of Medicine for the Care of Older People. (Clinical Directors)

Assessment of capacity and appropriate use of the consent process should be clearly understood and documented by all clinicians taking consent in the elderly. (Clinical Directors)

Medicine reviews need to be a regular daily occurrence in the peri-operative period. Input of both Medicine for the Care of Older People (MCOP) clinicians and an experienced ward pharmacist may greatly assist this process. (Clinical Directors)

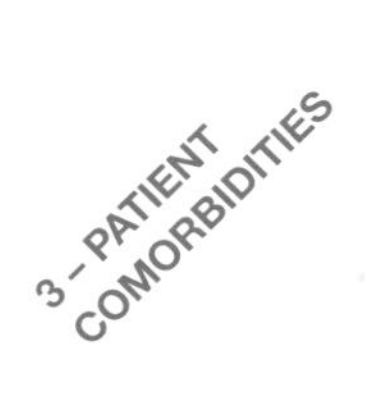


***References***


1. Office for National Statistics. 2001 Census. http://www.statistics.gov.uk/hub/health-social-care/index.html

2. Muravchick S. Pre-operative assessment of the elderly patient. *Anesthesiology Clinics North America.* 2000; 18, 71 - 89

3. National Institute for Clinical Excellence. *Preoperative testing- the use of routine preoperative tests for elective surgery*. 2003. www.nice.org.uk

4. Chandra SI. Systolic hypertension in older patients. *Journal of the American Medical Association*. 2004; 292, 1074 - 1080.

5. Schillinger M. Cardiovascular risk stratification in older patients. *Journal of the American Medical Association*. 2005; 293, 1667 - 1669.

6. Grobhan L & Butterworth J. Peri-operative management of chronic heart failure. *Anaesthesia and Analgesia.* 2006; 103(3), 557 - 575

7. Commission for Social Care Inspection, Audit Commission and Health Care Commission. *Living well in later life. A review of progress against the National Service Framework*. 2006. Commission for Healthcare Audit and Inspection.

8. Help the Aged. *Facts and figures about people around the world; July 2008*. 2008. http://www.helptheaged.org.uk/NR/rdonlyres/759CCFCC-911F-4AFC-9D1F-6F9C82BD993E/0/international_facts.pdf

9. Cook DJ & Rooke GA. Priorities in peri-operative geriatrics. Anaesthesia Analgesia. 2003; 96, 1823 - 1836

10. Charles Sturt University. *Frailty; a robust approach*. 2010. http://www.csu.edu.au/faculty/science/frailty/index.htm Last accessed 23rd August 2010.

11. Lally F & Crome P. Understanding frailty, *Postgraduate Medical Journal* 2007; 83, 16 - 20

12. Rockwood K, Howlett, SE et al. Prevalence, attributes and outcomes of fitness and frailty in community dwelling older adults: report from Canadian study of health and ageing. *Journals of Gerontology. Series A, Biological Sciences and Medical Sciences*. 2004; 591, 1310 - 1317

13. Rockwood K. What would make a definition of frailty successful? *Age and Ageing*. 2007; 34(5), 432 - 434

14. Rockwood K, Stadnyk K et al. A brief clinical instrument to classify frailty in elderly people. *The Lancet*. 1999; 353(9148), 205 - 206

15. Rockwood K, Song X, et al. A global clinical measure of fitness and frailty in elderly people. *Canadian Medical Journal*. 2005; 173,489-95

16. Fried LP, Tangen CM et al. Frailty in older adults. Evidence for a phenotype. *The Journals of Gerontology: Series A*. 2010; 56(3), M146 – M157

17. MacKay MA, Segev DL et al. Frailty as a predictor of surgical outcomes in older patients. *Journal of the American College of Surgeons*. 2010; 210, 901 - 908

18. World Health Organisation. *Nutritional Anaemias: Report of a WHO Group of Experts*. 1968. World Health Organisation. Geneva

19. Izaks GJ, Westerndorp RG & Knook DL. The definition of anaemia in older persons. *Journal of the American Medical Association*. 1999; 281, 1714 - 1717

20. Wu W, Schifftner TL et al. Preopertaive heamatocrit levels and post operative outcomes in older patients undergoing non cardiac surgery. *Journal of the American Medical Association*. 2007; 297(22), 2481 - 2488

21. Vincent JL, Baron J et al. Anaemia and blood transfusion in critically ill patients. *Journal of the American Medical Association.* 2002; 288(12), 1499 - 1507

22. Pederson T, Eliasen K & Henriksen E. A prospective study of risk factors and cardiopulmonary complications associated with anaesthesia and surgery:risk indicators of cardiopulmonary mortality. *Acta Anaesthesiologica Scandinavica*. 1990; 34, 144 - 155

23. National Confidential Enquiry into Patient Outcome and Death. *Extremes of Age, The 1999 report of the National Confidential Enquiry into Peri-operative Death.* 1999. NCEPOD, London

24. Department of Health & Philip I. *Better Health in Old Age.* 2004. Crown Copyright

25. The Patients Association. Incidence of hearing and visual loss in elderly. Patient.co.uk. Last accessed August 2010

26. Bracewell C, Gray R & RAI GS. *Essential Facts in Geriatric Medicine*. 2005 Radcliffe Publishing

27. National Institute for Clinical Excellence. Dementia-supporting people with dementia and their carers in health and social care. 2006. www.nice.org.uk

28. Scottish Intercollegiate Guidelines Network. *Managing patients with Dementia*. A National clinical guideline. 2006. Scottish Intercollegiate guidelines network. www.sign.ac.uk

29. Department of Health. *A National Dementia Strategy-Living well with dementia*. 2009. Crown Copyright

30. Royal College of Physicians. The Prevention, Diagnosis and Management of Delirium in Older People. National Guidelines. 2006. Royal College of Physicians

31. National Institute for Heath and Clinical Excellence Guidance. *Delirium: diagnosis, prevention and management.* 2010. National Institute for Clinical Health and Excellence.

32. Cashman J & Grounds M. Recent advances in Anaesthesia and Intensive Care 2007. Cambridge University Press

33. International Study of Post Operative Cognitive Dysfunction. http://www.sps.ele.tue.nl/ispocd/index.html Last updated 13 March 2006

34. Hanning CD. Post operative cognitive dysfunction. *British Journal of Anaesthesia*. 2005; 95(1), 82 - 87

35. Newman S, Stygall J et al. Post operative Cognitive Dysfunction after Noncardiac Surgery: A Systematic Review. *Anesthesiology*. 2007; 106(3), 572 - 590

36. Parker MJ, Handoll HHG, Griffiths R. *Anaesthesia for Hip fractures in adults. Cochrane systematic review.* 2004. The Cochrane Collaboration.

37. British Geriatrics Society & Royal College of Physicians. *Guidelines for the prevention, diagnosis and management of delirium in older people. Concise guidance to good practice series.* No. 6. 2006. Royal College of Physicians.

38. Fodale V, Quattrone D et al. Alzheimer's disease and anaesthesia: implications for the central cholinergic system. *British Journal of Anaesthesia. 2006*; 97(4), 445 - 452

39. British Geriatrics Society. *British Geriatrics Society Guidelines on capacity and testamentary capacity. Best Practice Guidance*. Updated March 2006. http://www.bgs.org.uk/Publications/Compendium/compend_2-2.htm Last accessed 28th September 2010

40. The Mental Capacity Act. 2005. Crown Copyright. http://www.legislation.gov.uk/ukpga/2005/9/contents

41. Department of Health. *Reference guide to consent for examination or treatment. 1st edition.* 2001. Crown Copyright

42. Department of Health. *Reference guide to consent for examination or treatment. 2nd edition*. 2009. Crown Copyright

43. Department of Health. *Seeking consent: working with older people*. 2001. Crown Copyright.

44. Department of Health. *The National Service Framework for older people*. 2001. Crown Copyright

45. Mallet L, Spinewine A & Huang A. The challenge of managing drug interactions in elderly people. *The Lancet*. 2007; 370, 185-191

46. Cooper N, Forrest K & Mulley G. ABC of *Geriatric Medicine.* 2009. Wiley-Blackwell.

47. Department of Health. *Medicines and older people-implementing medicines related aspects of the NSF for older people*. 2001. Crown Copyright

48. British Association of Parenteral and Enteric Nutrition. *Nutrition screening survey in UK 2007. A report by BAPEN. Nutrition screening survey and audit of adults on admission to hospitals, care homes and mental health units.* 2008. BAPEN

49. Ramaiah R & Lam AM. Post operative cognitive dysfunction in the elderly. *Anaesthesiology Clinics.* 2009; 27(3), 485 - 496

50. Milton JC, Hill-Smith I & Jackson SHD. Prescribing for older people. *British Medical Journal.* 2008; 336, 606-609

# 4 – Pre-operative care

Most surgery occurred in the context of acute illness and as an "urgent" or "emergency" event, the risks of which are known to be particularly high in this age group. The population had a large burden of co-morbidity, disability and frailty, as described in Chapter 3 and on admission 86% (915/1069) were classified using the American Society of Anaesthesiologists (ASA) score as ASA 3, 4 or 5 pre-operatively (143 were classified as ASA 1 or 2; in 65 cases this was not answered). Although the ASA grading was completed retrospectively at the time of completing the questionnaire this data nevertheless suggests that this population of elderly patients would have required careful pre-operative assessment before any procedure was undertaken.

## Admission and assessment process

In *Extremes of Age*,[1] the earlier NCEPOD classification of admission of Elective, Urgent and Emergency was used. 85% were classed as emergency, 7% as urgent, and 7% as elective. In the present study the majority of patients were also admitted as emergencies, but a slightly greater proportion of elective admissions were included (83.4% emergency, 14.1% elective, 2.4% planned (Chapter 1, Table 1.1).

In 1999, NCEPOD found that 54% of surgical patients over 90 years were admitted via the emergency department (ED) and 27% following referral from their general practitioner (GP). In the present study, a smaller percentage of patients aged 80 and over were admitted via their GP (17.9%) (Chapter 1, Table 1.2).

As in the previous study, the majority of elderly patients were ultimately managed by general (including sub specialty) surgeons or orthopaedic surgeons although the initial assessment was undertaken by Emergency Medicine in 37.1% (366/972) (Figure 4.1). This was not answered in 148 cases.

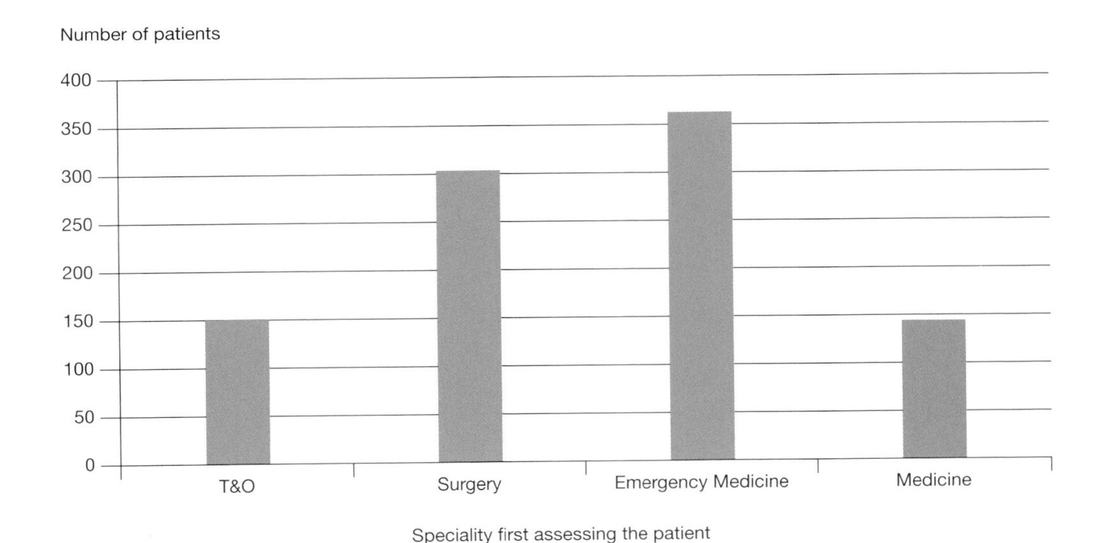


**Figure 4.1. Specialty of the healthcare professional responsible for the first assessment on arrival**

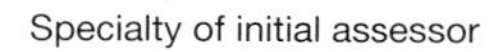

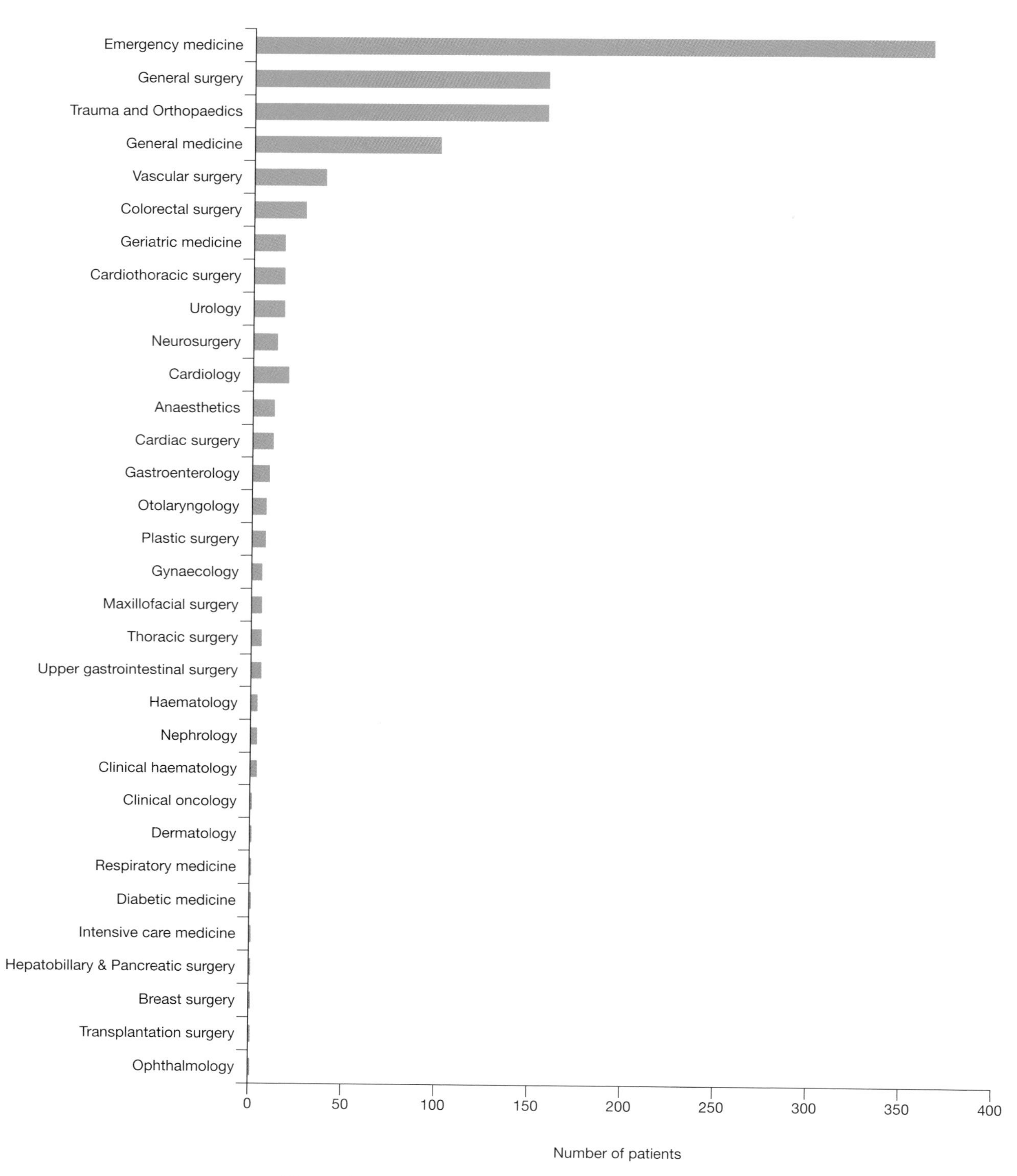


**Figure 4.2. Sub specialty of the healthcare professional responsible for first assessment on arrival**

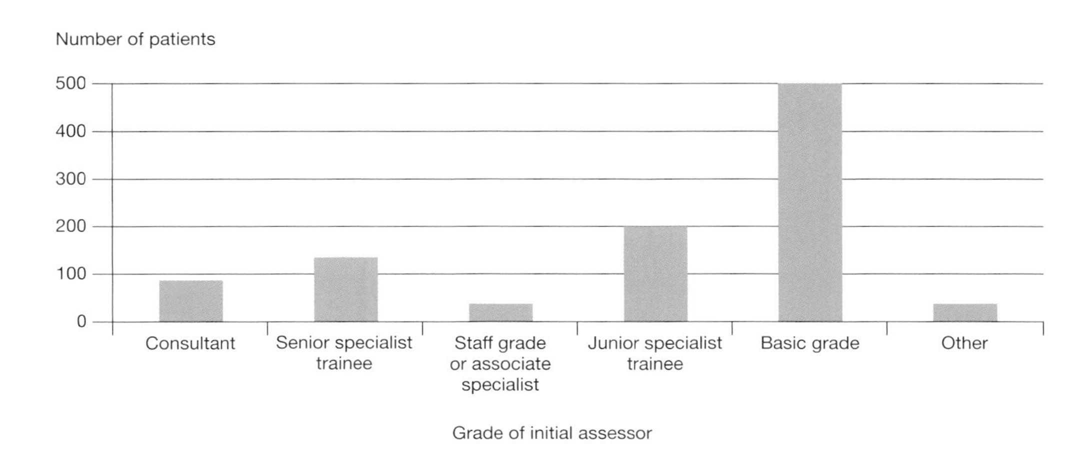


**Figure 4.3. Grade of the healthcare professional responsible for the first assessment**

All surgical sub-specialties (and some medical specialties) performed initial assessments of elderly patients on their arrival at hospital. Figure 4.2 gives a more detailed breakdown of these sub specialities.

Following admission, in 3.6% (40/1106) of cases the surgeons completing the questionnaires were of the opinion that the patient was initially admitted to the wrong specialty (1053/1106 were admitted to the appropriate specialty, and in 13/1106 cases it was unknown; it was not answered in 14 cases).

**Table 4.1 Admission to the most appropriate speciality – Advisors' opinion**

| Appropriate specialty | n | % |
|---|---|---|
| Yes | 741 | 92.7 |
| No | 58 | 7.3 |
| **Subtotal** | **799** | |
| Unable to answer | 20 | |
| Not answered | 1 | |
| **Total** | **820** | |

After review of the case notes Advisors were of the opinion that 58 patients were not admitted to the most appropriate specialty (Table 4.1); of these it was assessed that this had an adverse effect on outcome in 16 cases (no impact in 31, unable to answer in 6, and not answered in 5).

## Grade of healthcare professional responsible for the first assessment

The initial assessor in the ED was most often a basic grade doctor (Figure 4.3).

In a total of 694/992 cases basic and junior specialist trainees made the first assessment. It was unknown who made the first assessment in 128 cases.

Advisors were asked to make a global assessment of the appropriateness of the specialty and seniority of the clinician undertaking the initial assessment. In the majority of cases, Advisors were of the opinion that both the specialty and seniority of the first assessor were appropriate (Table 4.2).

Across the various specialties, there was considerable variation in the seniority of first assessor on arrival (Figure 4.4).

**Table 4.2 Appropriateness of the grade, time and specialty of the initial assessment for the severity and complexity of the illness or surgical condition – Advisors' opinion**

| Initial assessment appropriate | n | % |
|---|---|---|
| Yes | 714 | 95.8 |
| No | 31 | 4.2 |
| **Subtotal** | **745** | |
| Unable to answer | 69 | |
| Not answered | 6 | |
| **Total** | **820** | |

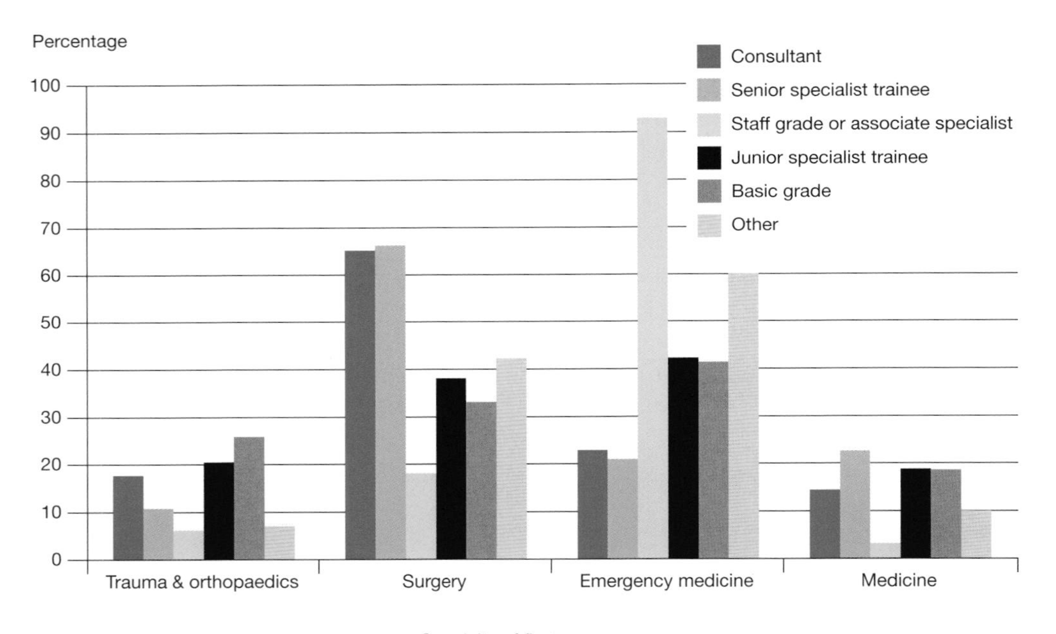


**Figure 4.4. Grade by specialty of the healthcare professional responsible for the first assessment on arrival**

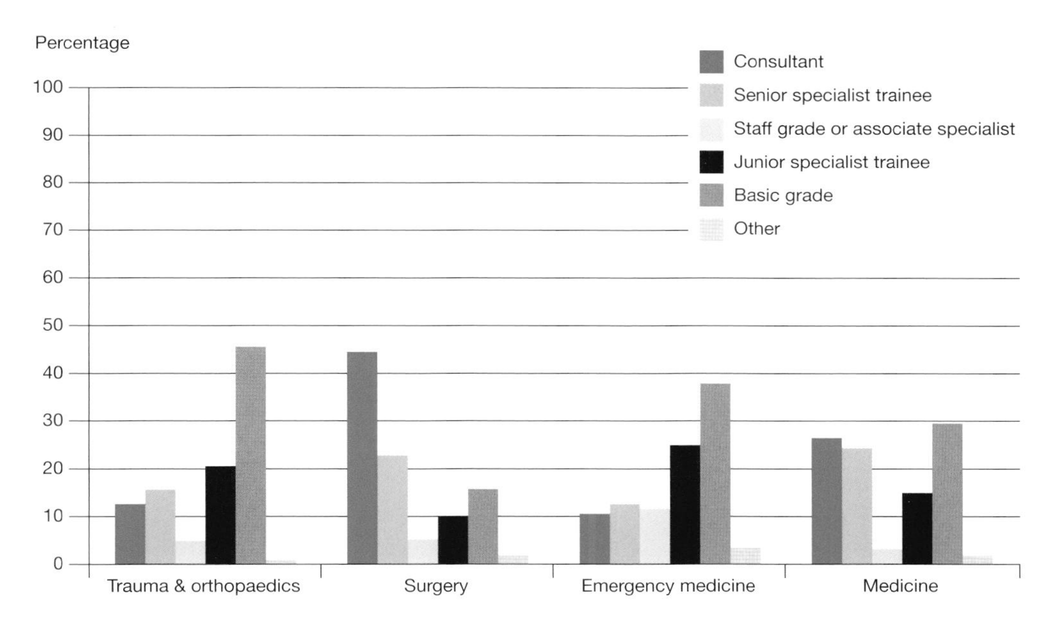


**Figure 4.5. Grade and specialty of the clinician deciding to admit the patient**

When the grade of doctor deciding to admit the patient is considered, a greater variation between the different specialties emerges, with a predominance of basic grade trainees being the most senior decision maker at this point of the care pathway for orthopaedics, emergency medicine and general medicine (Figure 4.5). This will be considered in more detail in the section relating to management of patients with fractured neck of femur.

There was some disagreement between Advisors in the different specialties, and in particular between Advisors in Trauma and Orthopaedic (T&O) surgery and Advisors in Medicine for the Care of Older People (MCOP). Many of the T&O Advisors were of the view that it was not inappropriate for the initial assessment to be made by basic grade orthopaedic doctors. MCOP Advisors thought that these complex elderly sick patients would benefit from early assessment of not only the surgical aspects of their health, but of their pre-existing comorbidities. The basic medical skills required to provide care of elderly patients should be well within the abilities of all junior doctors whether they are working in medicine, surgery or anaesthesia. Whilst symptoms and signs of disease may be less obvious in the elderly, and time may be required to identify them, it is essential that this information is properly sought at the first contact if the correct care pathways are then to be followed. Case study 6 on page 49 is an example of this.

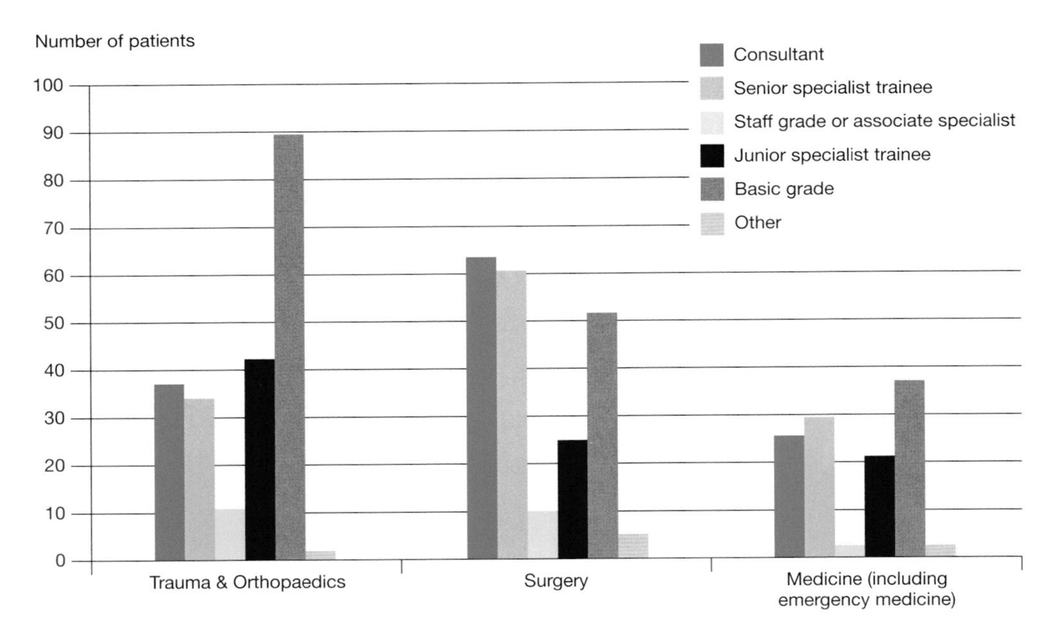


**Figure 4.6. Grade and specialty of first assessor following admission**

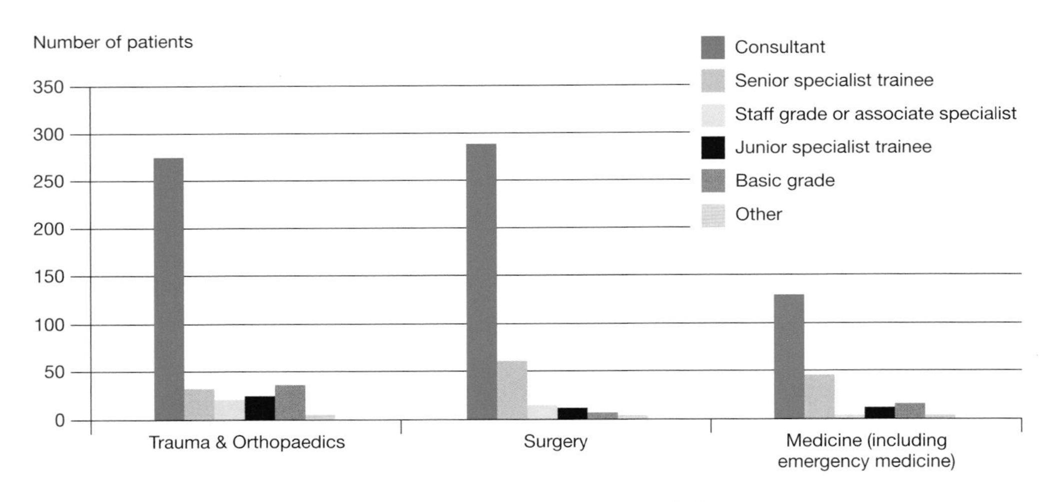


**Figure 4.7. Grade of clinician making the diagnosis by specialty of first assessor following admission**

## Assessment and diagnosis following specialty admission

Once admitted to hospital, the grade of clinician undertaking the subsequent assessment also varied considerably between the different specialties. Once again it can be seen that the majority of assessment in trauma and orthopaedics (T&O) are undertaken by basic grades (Figure 4.6). Case study 6 demonstrates an example of poor initial assessment.

However, when asked what grade of clinician made the diagnosis, there appears to be a much higher level of consultant involvement across the specialties (Figure 4.7).

**Case study 6**

A patient was admitted from the Emergency Department by a Foundation Year 2 covering urology. The patient was noted to be dehydrated with poor renal function, had a pelvic mass and there was reported per-vaginal bleeding. An abdominal and pelvic ultrasound scan was performed. Bilateral obstructed uropathy was diagnosed and a nephrostomy performed by the radiologist. Following the procedure the patient's condition deteriorated and after review by an anaesthetic Specialist Registrar was moved to a High Dependency Unit (HDU). When clerked on the HDU, the patient was noted to have a large carcinoma of the breast, and subsequent CT demonstrated widespread metastatic lesions.

*Advisors believed that there was a lack of basic medical skills, and failure to undertake a thorough physical examination by a number of junior trainees.*

In only 11.1% of cases was the diagnosis made by basic grades or junior trainees alone (Table 4.3).

**Table 4.3 Grade of the most senior healthcare professional making the diagnosis**

| Grade of clinician making the diagnosis | n | % |
|---|---|---|
| Consultant | 755 | 69.6 |
| Senior specialist trainee | 155 | 14.3 |
| Staff grade or associate specialist | 45 | 4.1 |
| Junior specialist trainee | 52 | 4.8 |
| Basic grade | 68 | 6.3 |
| Other | 10 | <1 |
| **Subtotal** | **1085** | |
| Not answered | 35 | |
| **Total** | **1120** | |

## Delays in assessment

Advisors' assessing the case notes were asked if there was any evidence of a delay in the patient being assessed by a consultant (Table 4.4).

**Table 4.4 Was there evidence of a delay in the patient being assessed by a consultant? – Advisor opinion**

| Delays in consultant review | n | % |
|---|---|---|
| Yes | 107 | 18.0 |
| No | 487 | 82.0 |
| **Subtotal** | **594** | |
| Unable to answer | 204 | |
| Not answered | 22 | |
| **Total** | **820** | |

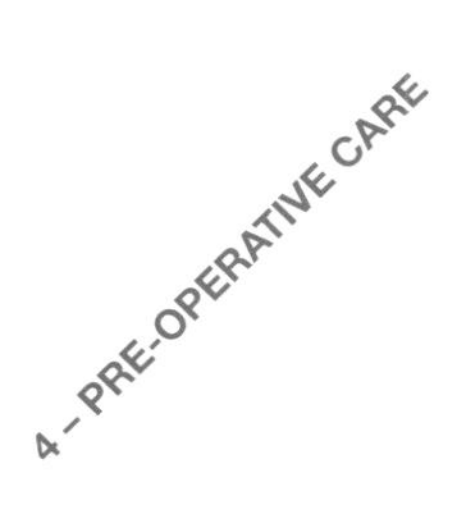


In nearly 1 in 5 patients where this could be determined there was a delay in assessment as judged by Advisors. This could have resulted in a further deterioration in the patients condition prior to treatment. The following case study demonstrates a delay in consultant review.

**Case study 7**

A patient attended the Emergency Department in the early hours of the morning and was eventually admitted mid morning with small bowel obstruction to a surgical ward. It was planned that an assessment by a surgical consultant would take place on the ward. However, the consultant was unable to assess the patient until 8pm because in addition to being on call they were undertaking an outpatient clinic and elective operating list. Despite laparotomy the next day, the patient succumbed to multi-organ failure.

*Advisors thought that had the consultant been available to review the patient promptly, the outcome might have been more favourable.*

## Decision to operate

In the majority of cases across all specialties, the decision to operate was taken by a consultant. Although the decision to admit and the initial assessment was often delegated to junior medical personnel, systems must be in place for early review by seniors to implement diagnostic and treatment plans.

The intended outcome of surgery was not always clear. Whilst in the majority of cases, the purpose of the operation was curative, in 14.2% it was regarded as palliative. In a number of cases, there were multiple intentions of surgery or the question was not answered (Table 4.5).

**Table 4.5 Treatment intention**

| Treatment intention | n | % |
|---|---|---|
| Diagnostic | 51 | 4.8 |
| Diagnostic and curative | 45 | 4.2 |
| Diagnostic and palliative | 17 | 1.6 |
| Diagnostic and curative and palliative | 3 | <1 |
| Curative | 780 | 73.4 |
| Curative and palliative | 15 | 1.4 |
| Palliative | 151 | 14.2 |
| **Subtotal** | **1062** | |
| Not answered | 58 | |
| **Total** | **1120** | |

The following case demonstrates an example of a lack of clarity of the purpose of the operation, and use of surgery without appropriate use of all available non-invasive diagnostic tests.

**Case study 8**

A patient was admitted with bowel obstruction having previously undergone a bowel resection 13 years previously for a Dukes C carcinoma. A laparotomy was performed with diagnostic/ palliative intent, by a consultant. At laparotomy, peritoneal deposits of carcinoma and liver metastases were discovered. Surgery lasted 4 hours, and post operatively the patient was sent to ICU and could not be weaned off the ventilator.

*Advisors questioned whether better pre-operative assessment and multi-disciplinary input might have permitted clearer treatment intent to have been established, and allowed palliation to be achieved by less invasive methods.*

**Table 4.6 Were there any delays – anaesthetist opinion**

| Reason for delay | Clinical | Organisational | Both clinical and organisational | Total delay | No delay (n) | Total |
|---|---|---|---|---|---|---|
| | Delay (n) | | | | | |
| The decision to operate | 135 | 31 | 42 | **208** | 749 | **957** |
| Pre-operative stabilisation | 111 | 6 | 18 | **135** | 822 | **957** |
| Obtaining routine testing | 20 | 5 | 11 | **36** | 921 | **957** |
| Obtaining specialist investigations | 26 | 15 | 9 | **50** | 907 | **957** |
| Obtaining a medical specialist opinion | 16 | 7 | 8 | **31** | 926 | **957** |
| Access to an operating theatre | 9 | 70 | 22 | **101** | 856 | **957** |
| Admission to HDU/ICU | 3 | 15 | 6 | **24** | 933 | **957** |
| Availability of a surgeon | 8 | 9 | 6 | **23** | 934 | **957** |
| Availability of an anaesthetist | 8 | 5 | 5 | **18** | 939 | **957** |
| Recovery | 2 | 1 | 5 | **8** | 949 | **957** |

## Urgency of operation

The majority of operations were classified as urgent according to the NCEPOD classification (Figure 4.8 see overleaf).

## Delays

According to the Anaesthetist completing the questionnaire there were 634 incidents of delays (answers could be multiple) and included decision to operate (208/957), pre-operative stabilisation (135/957), obtaining special investigations in 50/957 and access to an operating theatre in 101/957 (Table 4.6).

According to surgeons completing the questionnaire in 331/1081 cases they indicated that there was a delay between admission and surgery, (Table 4.7).

**Table 4.7 Delays between admission and operation**

| Delays between admission and operation | n | % |
|---|---|---|
| Yes | 331 | 30.6 |
| No | 737 | 68.2 |
| Unknown | 13 | 1.2 |
| **Subtotal** | **1081** | |
| Not answered | 39 | |
| **Total** | **1120** | |

Interpreting the cause of delay and in particular whether the delay was appropriate or justified is often difficult retrospectively.

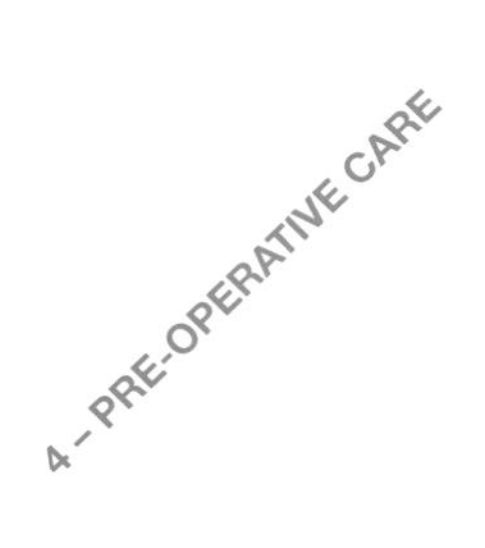


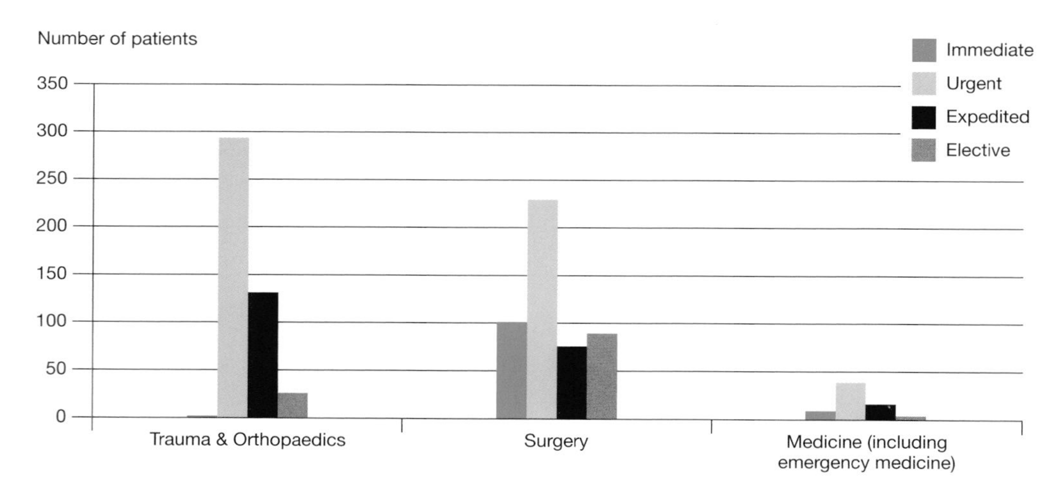


**Figure 4.8. Classification of urgency of operation by the specialty of the most senior clinician proposing the procedure**

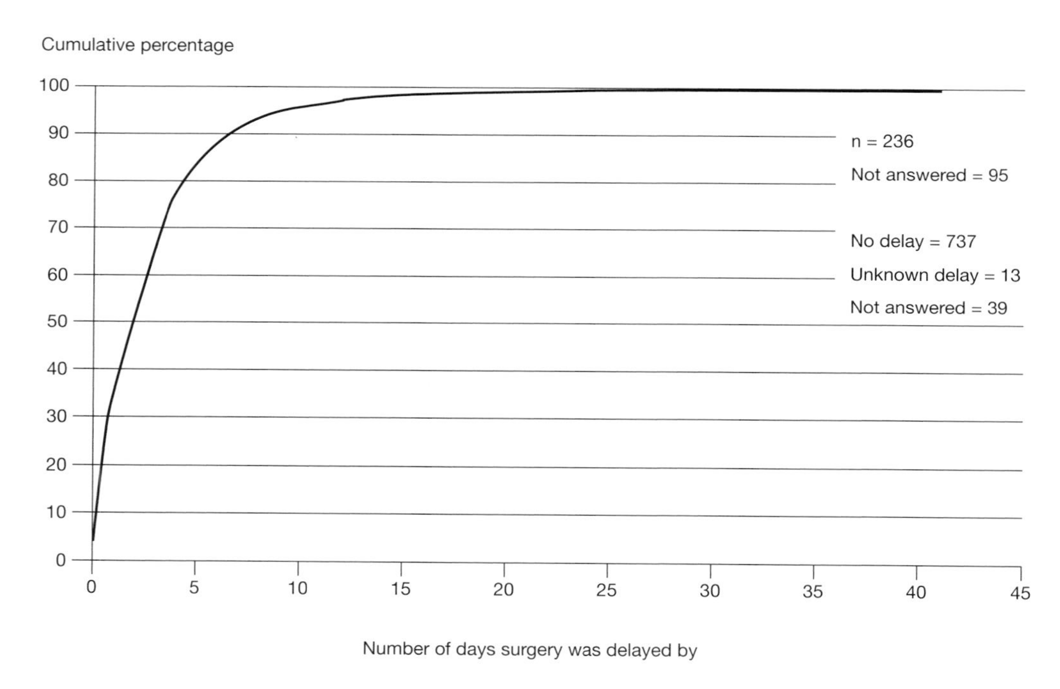


**Figure 4.9. Where there was a delay, how many days was surgery delayed by?**

### Length of delay

Surgeons completing the questionnaire were asked to quantify this delay. Surgery was delayed in 236 cases in total; where there was a delay this was by 1 day in 80 (33.9%) cases and by 2 days in 119 cases (50.4%) (Figure 4.9).

### Duration of delay between decision to operate and time of surgery – Advisors' opinion

In the 729 cases where both the surgical questionnaire and case notes were returned and it was possible to determine timings from the case notes, Advisors documented the times from the decision to operate from being declared ready for surgery and the induction of anaesthesia for urgent and emergency admissions. In 357/498 patients this was less than 24 hours, in 82 patients this was between 24 – 48 hours and in 59 patients this was greater than 48 hours. The duration between being declared fit for surgery and the induction of anaesthesia was not determined in 48 cases, was not applicable in 36 cases, and was not answered in 37 cases. This analysis does not include the 110 patients admitted on an elective basis.

Delay will be examined in more detail specifically for those patients undergoing surgery for an acute abdomen and fractured neck of femur.

Advisors were also asked to identify on a case by case basis, whether an operation had been completed in a timely manner without significant delay (Table 4.8).

**Table 4.8 Operation performed in a timely manner – Advisors' opinion**

| Operation performed in a timely manner | n | % |
|---|---|---|
| Yes | 615 | 75.6 |
| No | 174 | 21.4 |
| **Subtotal** | **814** | |
| Unable to answer | 25 | |
| Not answered | 6 | |
| **Total** | **820** | |

Clinically significant delay was deemed to have occurred in 21% of cases by the Advisors. This was one of the major recurring themes identified as a contributory factor to less than good care by the Advisors.

### Expectation of survival

**Table 4.9 Expectation of survival of the patient**

| Expectation of survival | n | % |
|---|---|---|
| Yes | 573 | 52.6 |
| No | 121 | 11.1 |
| Unknown | 395 | 36.3 |
| **Subtotal** | **1089** | |
| Not answered | 31 | |
| **Total** | **1120** | |

Surgeons completing the questionnaire expected just over half of the patients to survive their admission (Table 4.9). They believed death to be the likely outcome in 11%, but in 36% of cases they were uncertain.

Predicting death is notoriously difficult even for the most experienced clinicians and this highlights the problem of establishing a treatment plan which is appropriate and in the best interests of the patient in a timely manner. The likelihood of an appropriate and timely treatment plan being established is enhanced if the skill and experience of the clinicians is appropriate to the severity of illness of the patient. In over half of those patients not expected to survive, an operation was performed with curative intent whilst in 20.2% of cases the operation was considered palliative (Table 4.10).

**Table 4.10 Operative intent by expectation of survival**

| | Expected to survive | | | | | | | | |
|---|---|---|---|---|---|---|---|---|---|
| | Yes | | No | | Unknown | | Subtotal | Not answered | Total |
| **Operative intent** | **n** | **%** | **n** | **%** | **n** | **%** | **n** | **n** | **n** |
| Diagnostic | 16 | 2.9 | 12 | 10.5 | 21 | 5.6 | **49** | 2 | **51** |
| Diagnostic and Curative | 17 | 3.1 | 10 | 8.8 | 17 | 4.5 | **44** | 1 | **45** |
| Diagnostic and Curative and Palliative | 1 | 0.2 | 0 | 0.0 | 1 | 0.3 | **2** | 1 | **3** |
| Diagnostic and Palliative | 5 | 0.9 | 3 | 2.6 | 9 | 2.4 | **17** | 0 | **17** |
| Curative | 440 | 80.7 | 65 | 57.0 | 260 | 68.8 | **765** | 15 | **781** |
| Curative and Palliative | 8 | 1.5 | 1 | 0.9 | 6 | 1.6 | **15** | 0 | **15** |
| Palliative | 58 | 10.6 | 23 | 20.2 | 64 | 16.9 | **145** | 6 | **151** |
| **Subtotal** | **545** | | **114** | | **378** | | **1037** | **25** | **1062** |
| Not answered | 28 | | 7 | | 17 | | **52** | 6 | **58** |
| **Total** | **573** | | **121** | | **395** | | **1089** | **31** | **1120** |

It should be highlighed that 17 of the patients in the group not expected to survive underwent a minor procedure, for example a feeding gastrostomy.

**Table 4.11 Changes in ASA status between admission and operation**

| | | Health status prior to surgery (n) | | | | | | | |
|---|---|---|---|---|---|---|---|---|---|
| | | ASA 1 | ASA 2 | ASA 3 | ASA 4 | ASA 5 | **Subtotal** | Not answered | **Total** |
| **Health status on admission (n)** | ASA 1 | 3 | 0 | 0 | 0 | 0 | **3** | 0 | **3** |
| | ASA 2 | 1 | 123 | 11 | 3 | 1 | **139** | 1 | **140** |
| | ASA 3 | 0 | 22 | 449 | 14 | 1 | **486** | 9 | **495** |
| | ASA 4 | 0 | 13 | 65 | 289 | 4 | **371** | 2 | **373** |
| | ASA 5 | 0 | 4 | 14 | 8 | 20 | **46** | 1 | **47** |
| | **Subtotal** | **4** | **162** | **539** | **314** | **26** | **1045** | **13** | **1058** |
| | Not answered | 0 | 8 | 12 | 17 | 3 | **40** | 22 | **62** |
| | **Total** | **4** | **163** | **548** | **316** | **27** | **1085** | **35** | **1120** |

## ASA status and expectation of survival

We have already noted the large burden of comorbidity in this population which was broadly reflected in ASA status on admission, with 84% (879/1045) falling in the ASA groups 3, 4 and 5 (Table 1.3, Chapter 1). There were small changes (both improvement and deterioration) in status between admission and operation, (Table 4.11). As noted earlier, these scores were derived retrospectively.

## Risk stratification

As well as ASA scoring there are systems in use which may provide better risk stratification of patients prior to surgery, and thus plan best care. These include cardiopulmonary exercise testing (CPX) and both formal and informal severity scoring. CPX testing has been applied most successfully to elective patients for major bowel resection.[2,3,4] Most of the patients in this study underwent urgent or emergency surgery and so these tests would not usually have been applicable.

Nevertheless we asked anaesthetists whether, if the patient had been seen in a pre-assessment clinic, if any formal assessment of cardiopulmonary reserve had been made (Table 4.12). In very few instances was this the case.

**Table 4.12 Formal pre-operative assessment of cardiopulmonary reserve if the patient was seen at an anaesthetic pre-assessment clinic.**

| Assessment of cardiopulmonary reserve | n |
|---|---|
| Yes | 16 |
| No | 59 |
| Unknown | 3 |
| **Subtotal** | **78** |
| Not answered | 2 |
| **Total** | **80** |

However, whilst 115/157 elective patients attended traditional Pre-Assessment Clinic (PAC), only 16 seemed to have their management altered, (89 did not have their management altered, it was unknown in 4 cases and not answered in 6). If the facility had been available it may well be that CPX would have provided a more specific method of providing targeted management to those patients undergoing major surgery.[5] Most studies to date are in patients undergoing abdominal surgery.[6,7,8,9] Surrogates that could also guide management in the emergency setting need to be considered.

It may also be that traditional severity scores require modification for the elderly as they do not fully take into account additional factors such as frailty, and level of preoperative disability, both of which will influence survival, and the ability to leave hospital and return to independent function. More recent scoring systems[10] weight existing indices to improve prediction in the elderly. It should be stressed that such scoring systems are useful primarily in the context of analysing populations and cannot be used to make individual treatment decisions.

In the opinion of our Advisors, and in the absence of other bedside "tools", the input of experienced clinicians at an early stage remains a very important intervention in the elderly surgical population, and assists in the quantification of risk and the delivery of an appropriate level of care.

## Input from Medicine for the Care of Older People

As indicated above the health of these elderly patients on admission was poor (ASA grades 3-4). The patients presenting to the general surgeons were sicker and represented the majority of ASA 4 and 5 patients.

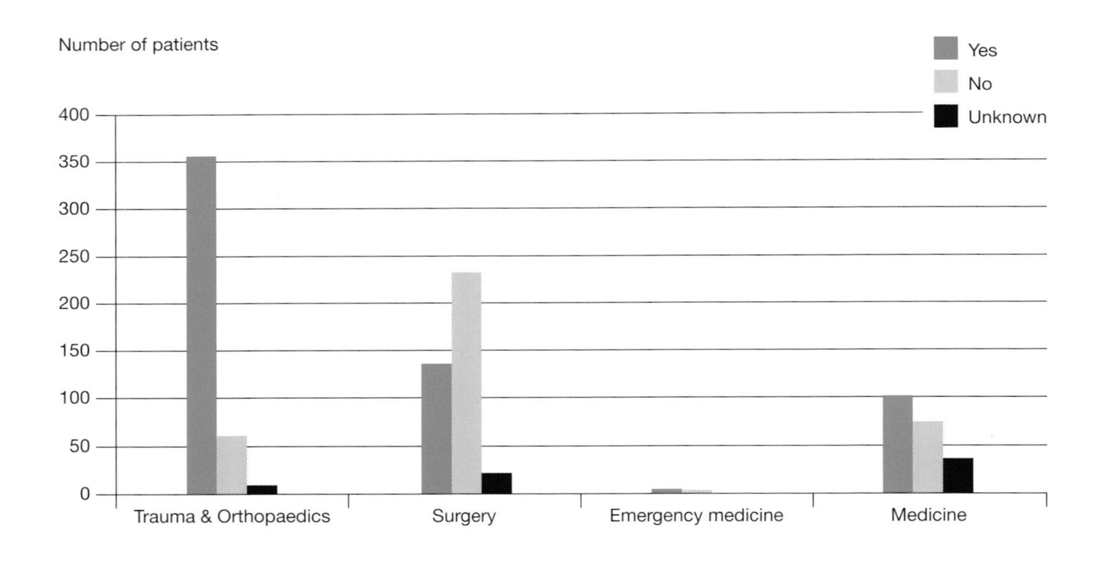


**Figure 4.10. Specialty of clinician the patient was first admitted to by formal input from MCOP to the surgical team**

There was a marked difference in MCOP input between patients admitted under T&O as compared to other surgical specialties (Figure 4.10). The majority (359/429) of patients admitted under T&O were said to have received some level of formal MCOP involvement pre and or post operatively. This could be explained, by the greater level of funded MCOP sessions in T&O, and by the requirements set out in the National Service Framework (NSF) for older people. It begs the question however, should elderly general surgical patients also have formal input from MCOP specialists?

## Discussion at a Multidisciplinary Team (MDT) meeting

**Table 4.13 Case discussed at a MDT meeting prior to the operation**

| Case discussed at MDT meeting | n | % |
|---|---|---|
| Yes | 253 | 23.5 |
| No | 779 | 72.3 |
| Unknown | 46 | 4.3 |
| **Subtotal** | **1078** | |
| Not answered | 42 | |
| **Total** | **1120** | |

Less than a quarter of patients were formally considered in an MDT (Table 4.13), and whilst urgency may have often precluded this, there were occasions when it was clear that multidisciplinary input was both timely and indicated. Case study 9 presents an example of this.

**Case study 9**

An insulin dependent patient who had had previous strokes, had multi-infarct dementia, and chronic kidney disease was admitted from the surgical outpatient clinic with an ischaemic leg, and taken to theatre later that day for an above knee amputation. There was no involvement of MCOP, and no evidence of formal pre-operative anaesthetic assessment. Documentation was poor. The patient's diabetes was poorly managed, and there was no evidence in the notes that an appropriate consenting process had been undertaken.

*Advisors believed that mutli-disciplinary input would have led to the patient being better optimized before surgery and that both clinical and organisational aspects of care were very poor.*

The 2001 NSF for older people[11] recognised that care of the elderly in hospital is complex. It recommends that older people be given the early supervision and advice of a specialist team when admitted to an acute general hospital. In particular it states that there should be involvement of a consultant in old age medicine or rehabilitation, so that appropriate treatment and management decisions are made. As well as medical consultants who care for the elderly, specialist nurses/ nurse consultants, physiotherapists, occupational therapists and speech and language specialists, dieticians, social workers and care managers, and pharmacists are required.

The previous NCEPOD report on the elderly emphasised the importance of team working, and the involvement of the appropriate level of clinician, in terms of seniority and experience, in the care of the patients who have poor physical status and high operative risk.

# Pre-optimisation

## Overall pre-operative patient optimisation

In the opinion of Advisors whilst 606/717 patients had their condition adequately optimised pre-operatively, 111 did not. Advisors were unable to answer this question, or did not answer this question in 103 cases. Advisors indicated that involvement of MCOP clinicians could have improved the health status of some patients (52/103). Other recommended measures were fluid resuscitation (49/103), correction of electrolyte or blood sugar imbalance (26/103), or correction of anaemia (15/103), (answers may be multiple; not answered in 8 cases).

In the elderly patient presenting for surgery the risk of consequent serious morbidity and death are high. Pre-operative optimisation must be undertaken in a timely fashion in order to influence outcome, and this involves input from senior clinicians as part of a multidisciplinary team.

It was also expected that essential investigations and procedures to improve readiness for theatre should have been undertaken in this population.

**Table 4.14 All essential investigations required in preparation for surgery were performed – Advisors' opinion**

| Essential investigations performed | n | % |
|---|---|---|
| Yes | 693 | 90.7 |
| No | 71 | 9.3 |
| **Subtotal** | **764** | |
| Unable to answer | 53 | |
| Not answered | 3 | |
| **Total** | **820** | |

**Table 4.15 Clinical outcome affected by deficiencies in investigations – Advisors' opinion**

| Deficiencies in investigations effect on outcome | n | % |
|---|---|---|
| Yes | 75 | 12.2 |
| No | 541 | 87.8 |
| **Subtotal** | **616** | |
| Unable to answer | 72 | |
| Not answered | 132 | |
| **Total** | **820** | |

Advisors indicated that all essential investigations were performed in preparation for surgery in > 90% of patients (Table 4.14). In 276/793 patients investigations of an invasive nature were undertaken, (Advisors were unable to answer or did not answer in 27 cases). Overall there were deficiencies in pre-operative investigations in 71/764 patients (Table 4.14) and deficiencies in investigations were sufficient to affect outcome in 75/616 cases (Table 4.15). However looking specifically at the 71 patients where Advisors indicated that not all essential investigations had been performed, it was indicated this had a clinically significant effect on outcome in 34 cases, (no effect in 15 cases, unable to answer in 21 and did not answer in 1).

## Pre-assessment clinics

As the majority of patients involved in this study were admitted as emergencies, pre-assessment clinics did not feature prominently in the management of the patients in this study.

Table 4.16 Assessment in a pre-assessment clinic

| Attendance at a pre-assessment clinic | n | % |
|---|---|---|
| Yes | 122 | 11.6 |
| No | 909 | 86.7 |
| Unknown | 17 | 1.6 |
| **Subtotal** | **1048** | |
| Not answered | 72 | |
| **Total** | **1120** | |

Of the 122 patients who were assessed in a pre-assessment clinic (Table 4.16), only one was planned admission and 5 were emergencies. The remainder were elective admissions. Only 17 underwent therapeutic manoeuvres as a result of their pre-assessment (91 no, 5 unknown, 9 not answered). On only 3 occasions were discrepancies in the condition of the patient observed between pre-assessment and admission (108 no, 6 unknown, 5 not answered).

Of the 157 elective admissions there were 42 who were not seen in a PAC. The Advisors indicated that some of these would have benefited from pre-assessment, as this would have provided the opportunity to identify comorbidities, and optimise the physical status of patients prior to surgery. Case study 10 details such an example.

**Case study 10**

A patient was seen in a Head and Neck Cancer MDT with an advanced carcinoma of the cheek. Multiple comorbidities were present, including ischaemic heart disease, atrial fibrillation, diabetes, chronic kidney disease and obesity. The patient was on multiple medications. After considering radical surgery or radiotherapy the patient elected to have surgery; they did not attend a pre-assessment clinic, and on admission the diabetes and renal function had not been optimized. The patient developed Clostridium Difficile diarrhoea in the post operative period, and died 5 days later.

*Advisors were of the view that the patient would have benefited from pre-assessment and optimisation of physical status prior to surgery.*

## Anaesthetic pre-operative assessment

In more than 97% of cases there had been a pre-operative anaesthetic assessment (Table 4.17).

Table 4.17 Did an anaesthetist make a pre-operative assessment of the patient before the operation

| Anaesthetic pre-assessment | n | % |
|---|---|---|
| Yes | 928 | 97.5 |
| No | 21 | 2.2 |
| Unknown | 3 | 0.3 |
| **Subtotal** | **952** | |
| Not answered | 5 | |
| **Total** | **957** | |

In 64.5% of cases (613/951), the anaesthetist stated that they had been involved in the decision to operate, (not involved in 304 cases; it was unknown in 34 cases and not answered in 6 cases). In 95.2% (906/952) of cases they agreed that it was the correct decision to operate. They disagreed in 22 patients, it was unknown in 24 cases and the question was not answered in 5 instances. If assessed by an anaesthetist pre-operatively, we examined whether the same anaesthetist was present at the start of the operation. In 820/919 cases (89%) the pre-assessing anaesthetist was present at the start of the case, (no in 90 cases, unknown in 9 cases and not answered in 9 cases). Whilst it may not be practical to always have the same anaesthetist present during a case, it is important that both a verbal and written handover of patients takes place.[12]

### Optimisation of nutritional status

The correction of malnutrition has been shown to have effects on morbidity, mortality, length of hospital stay and wound healing.[13] Innovations such as the Organisation of Food and Nutritional Support in Hospitals (OFNOSH) initiative[14] and the red tray scheme[15] have been introduced to hospitals in an attempt to improve the nutritional status of inpatients.

It should be remembered that the majority of admissions within this study were emergencies. Whilst, at first glance, nutritional assessment may appear peripheral to other clinical activity during an emergency surgical admission, it is arguable that it is core to both post operative recovery and long term prognosis.

Surgeons completing the questionnaire reported that 93/967 (9.6%) (153 not answered) patients had malnutrition on admission. However just 55 of these were given nutritional support, 22 were not, in 15 cases it was unknown and not answered in 1 case. Furthermore, clinicians completing the questionnaire reported that only 206/1074 patients had a nutritional assessment (599 patients did not, in 269 patients it was unknown and in 46 not answered). However for 369/967 patients their nutritional status on admission could not be commented on, presumably owing to a lack of documentation (153 not answered). It is important to reiterate here however that on review (Table 3.2 Chapter 3), Advisors noted from both questionnaires and case notes that there was recognition of poor nutrition by the admitting team in 304/536 cases.

Only 118/721 patients had height, and 212/730 weight, recorded in the notes during their admission (Table 4.18). The predictable corollary of this being that just 99/723

**Table 4.18 Recording of height, weight and BMI in the case notes**

| Recorded in the case notes | Height | | Weight | | BMI | |
|---|---|---|---|---|---|---|
| | n | % | n | % | n | % |
| Yes | 118 | 16.4 | 212 | 29.0 | 99 | 13.7 |
| No | 603 | 83.6 | 518 | 71.0 | 624 | 86.3 |
| **Subtotal** | **721** | | **730** | | **723** | |
| Unable to answer | 96 | | 87 | | 92 | |
| Not answered | 3 | | 3 | | 5 | |
| **Total** | **820** | | **820** | | **820** | |

patients had their body mass index (BMI) calculated. The difficulties of measuring height in an acutely unwell elderly patient are considerable and with this in mind the low figure here is probably understandable. However, weight is an easier parameter to measure and is a clinical indicator of well being, vital in recording the response to nutritional therapy, and in the calculation of some drug dosages. That it was so low in this group of patients is of concern.

If patients are admitted to care homes it is a national recommendation that nutritional screening is undertaken, a record of weight maintained and appropriate action taken if patients are under or over weight.[16] When patients are admitted to hospital, this information, along with details of their medical problems should be sought from the patient and carers and referral notes constructed with as much information as possible from primary providers.

### Skin viability

Among other aspects of care the NSF drew attention to the importance of pressure sore risk management. However from the surgical questionnaire, it would appear that the assessment of skin viability is not always being documented or at least not documented where the surgeon can identify it easily (Table 4.19).

**Table 4.19 Assessment of skin viability**

| Skin viability assessed | n | % |
|---|---|---|
| Yes | 520 | 51.1 |
| No | 143 | 14.0 |
| Unknown | 355 | 34.9 |
| **Subtotal** | **1018** | |
| Not answered | 102 | |
| **Total** | **1120** | |

In *Extremes of Age*[1] it was noted that pressure sores were a frequent complication, particularly in orthopaedic patients. Since that publication, NICE has provided specific guidance on the avoidance of this complication[17] and thus routine assessment of risk should occur on admission.

### Optimisation of fluid balance and assessment of acute kidney injury

In 1999 a key recommendation of the *Extremes of Age* report was "fluid management in the elderly is often poor; it should be accorded the same status as drug prescription. Multidisciplinary reviews to develop good working practices are required".[1] In addition a recent report by NCEPOD *Adding Insult to Injury* has highlighted concerns regarding the recognition of acute kidney injury (AKI).[18] Elderly patients are at particular risk of AKI as glomerular filtration rate declines with age. When coupled with a surgical insult this may precipitate AKI.

**Table 4.20 Evidence of AKI being noted on admission – Advisors' opinion**

| AKI on admission | n | % |
|---|---|---|
| Yes | 186 | 24.3 |
| No | 579 | 75.7 |
| **Subtotal** | **765** | |
| Unable to answer | 48 | |
| Not answered | 7 | |
| **Total** | **820** | |

Based on case note review approximately a quarter of the patients (186/765) in this study had evidence of AKI on admission (Table 4.20). Furthermore there was clinical evidence of dehydration pre-operatively in 252/761 patients. This is unsurprising in an elderly population with surgical comorbidity.

Despite this, a third of patients (296/918) did not have any formal assessment of pre-operative fluid status (498 did, unknown in 163 cases) and a quarter of patients (156/609) did not have adequate assessment of other risk factors for developing, or having developed AKI (Table 4.21); furthermore pre-operative fluid resuscitation was assessed by Advisors as inadequate in 71/549 patients (Table 4.22). The elderly are a vulnerable group of patients whose renal function may already be compromised before the clinical emergency and/or surgery has occurred. Indeed following admission, the incidence of AKI rose further (248/678) probably reflecting declining renal function secondary to an ongoing surgical insult (this number includes 74 patients where AKI was noted on admission and they went on to develop AKI post admission) (In 142 cases the Advisors were unable to answer this.

In this study anaesthetists noted that in only 498/918 (54.2%) patients was there a record made of pre-operative hydration status; and perhaps worse there was no record in 296. This was in the context of cases showing 277/920 evidence of dehydration pre-operatively (no evidence in 573, unknown in 107 patients). In only 371/912 patients was there a record of pre-operative urine output, there being no record in 436, (unknown in 150 cases). A total of 415/927 patients required fluids to resuscitate them, and 122/925 patients received pre-operative blood or blood products.

**Table 4.21 Adequate assessment of the risk factors for AKI performed – Advisors' opinion**

| Adequate assessment of risk factors | n | % |
|---|---|---|
| Yes | 453 | 74.4 |
| No | 156 | 25.6 |
| **Subtotal** | **609** | |
| Unable to answer | 161 | |
| Not answered | 50 | |
| **Total** | **820** | |

**Table 4.22 Categorisation of pre-operative fluid resuscitation in acute admissions – Advisors' opinion**

| Pre-operative fluid resuscitation | n | % |
|---|---|---|
| Adequate/appropriate | 467 | 85.1 |
| Inadequate | 71 | 12.9 |
| Excessive | 11 | 2.0 |
| **Subtotal** | **549** | |
| Unable to answer | 116 | |
| Not applicable | 92 | |
| Not answered | 63 | |
| **Total** | **820** | |

The following case illustrates a number of points including the difficulties of achieving optimal fluid balance in patients with complex comorbidity.

**Case study 11**

A patient was admitted with a fractured NOF. They had IHD, COPD and pre-operatively was managed by junior orthopaedic trainees, without consultant or MCOP input. The patient oscillated between dehydration and fluid overload before undergoing an operation 6 days after admission. In the post operative period they developed pulmonary oedema and pneumonia. There was no evidence of senior input into their post operative care.

*Advisors felt that whilst surgery had been delayed because of complicating comorbidity, little had been done to improve the patients medical condition. Whilst the operation was straight forward, little was done to prevent post operative complications.*

## Pre-operative pain management

It is recognised that inadequate pain relief increases the risk of an adverse peri-operative outcome in the elderly by contributing to tachycardia, hypertension, cardiac ischaemia and hypoxemia. Effective analgesia can decrease the incidence of myocardial ischemia and pulmonary complications, accelerate recovery, promote early mobilisation, shorten hospital stay and reduce medical care costs. Poorly managed pain is also a risk factor for other complications in the elderly such as skin ulceration. Elderly patients may be more likely to under report the experience of pain, and may have very different ways of articulating their symptoms and needs. Communication problems make it more difficult for pain to be conveyed and understood by carers, particularly if the carers are unfamiliar with the patient.[19] Elderly patients may also have difficulty utilising standard methods of pain relief e.g. visual problems or reduced strength/mobility to operate patient controlled analgesia pumps. Pain is sometimes managed inadequately in the elderly for fear of overdose and respiratory depression.[20,21,22]

The 1999 NCEPOD report[1] found that pain management in the peri-operative period was often deficient and a key recommendation was that:
*"Elderly patients need their pain management to be provided by those with appropriate specialised experience in order that they receive safe and effective pain relief"*

The NSF for older people[11] commented specifically on poor pain management in the elderly. Patient groups have also pointed to deficiencies in attention to pain relief in the elderly.[23] Recently guidance has been published with regard to the assessment and management of pain in older people.[19]

## Initial pain assessment and early management

Chronic pain is more common in all elderly patients[24]. It has been estimated that > 50% of patients in a community setting and > 80% in a nursing home have persistent or chronic pain.[22] We expected that any initial health assessment in the elderly would aim to identify pain as a routine part of that consultation.[19]

Advisors were asked to judge whether pain had been assessed on admission. They could only be sure this had occurred in 520/641 cases. In 63 cases it was judged that pain assessment was inappropriate or unnecessary (Table 4.23).

**Table 4.23 Assessment of pain on admission – Advisors' opinion**

| Pain assessed on admission | n | % |
|---|---|---|
| Yes | 520 | 81.1 |
| No | 121 | 18.9 |
| **Subtotal** | **641** | |
| Inappropriate or unnecessary | 63 | |
| Unable to answer | 109 | |
| Not answered | 7 | |
| **Total** | **820** | |

Given that most admissions were for urgent or emergency surgery, pain was particularly likely to be a significant feature in these cases, but in 121 instances Advisors indicated pain was not assessed. Whilst in a small percentage of patients urgent life saving surgery was required, there is no excuse for not assessing and managing pain alongside resuscitation i.e. pain assessment and management is as essential in this context as recording pulse, blood pressure and oxygen saturation. The mode of admission was looked at in more detail and in 89/501 cases admitted as an emergency pain did not appear to have been assessed pre-operatively (Figure 4.11).

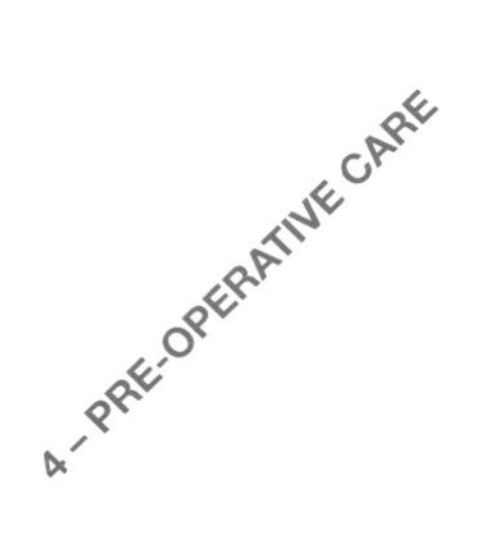


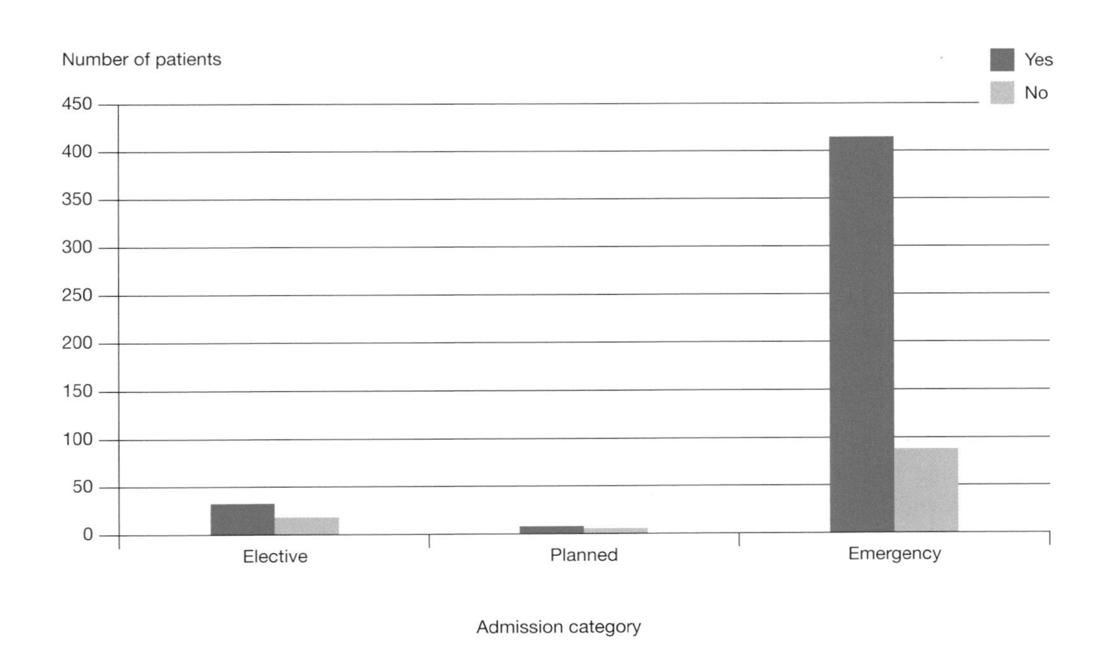


**Figure 4.11. Pain assessed on admission by category of admission**

Anaesthetists completing the questionnaire were also asked in the case of emergency surgery if they were aware whether patients had received analgesia pre-operatively. Of the 581 patients undergoing emergency surgery 79/556 had not received preoperative analgesia (Table 4.24).

**Table 4.24 Receipt of pre-operative analgesia in emergency surgery**

| Pre-operative analgesia | n | % |
|---|---|---|
| Yes | 446 | 80.2 |
| No | 79 | 14.2 |
| Unknown | 31 | 5.6 |
| **Subtotal** | **556** | |
| Not answered | 25 | |
| **Total** | **581** | |

Advisors were also asked to assess whether appropriate analgesia had been administered prior to surgery and were of the opinion that this was not the case in 41 patients (Table 4.25).

**Table 4.25 Appropriateness of analgesia given to the patient on admission and prior to surgery – Advisors' opinion**

| Appropriate analgesia administered | n | % |
|---|---|---|
| Yes | 467 | 91.9 |
| No | 41 | 8.1 |
| **Subtotal** | **508** | |
| Not answered | 21 | |
| Unable to answer | 174 | |
| Not applicable | 117 | |
| **Total** | **820** | |

It is now 20 years since a joint working party of the Royal College of Surgeons (RCS) and Royal College of Anaesthetist (RCoA) recommended consistent access to pain relief before and after surgery.[25] The lack of pain assessment and administration of analgesia is lamentable in this most vulnerable of populations.

## Involvement of pain teams pre-operatively

Anaesthetists completing the questionnaire were also asked whether patients had been referred to an acute pain team preoperatively; just 19% of patients had been referred (Table 4.26).

**Table 4.26 Referral of the patient to an acute pain team**

| Referral to an acute pain team | n | % |
|---|---|---|
| Yes | 175 | 18.9 |
| No | 620 | 67.0 |
| Unknown | 131 | 14.1 |
| **Subtotal** | **926** | |
| Not answered | 31 | |
| **Total** | **957** | |

Whilst it would be impractical to suggest that all patients should be seen by an Acute Pain Service (APS), protocols and guidelines should be in place to appropriately assess and manage pain. It has already been noted that 50-80% of elderly patients may have chronic pain on admission to hospital. Patients with severe ongoing chronic pain are best dealt with by input from pain specialists who will be more familiar with the sometimes complex regimens that are used to manage this and the potential for drug interactions. However it is recognised that an APS was not available in all Trusts and further data about this is presented in Chapter 6.

## Key findings

Risk assessment may be particularly difficult in the elderly surgical population, and should include input from senior surgeons, anaesthetists and Medicine for the Care of Older People (MCOP) clinicians.

A clinically significant delay between admission and operation occurred in over 1 in 5 elderly patients in this study (174/814), and is one of the major remediable factors identified by Advisors.

Malnutrition is common in elderly surgical admissions, but documentation, nutritional assessment and evidence of appropriate management within this group was extremely poor.

Acute kidney injury at the time of admission was an important cause of comorbidity in this elderly population (186/765) before surgery within this sample.

Pain was poorly assessed and documented. Pre-operative pain management in some patients was absent or inadequate in this sample.

## Recommendations

Delays in surgery for the elderly are associated with poor outcome. They should be subject to regular and rigorous audit in all surgical specialities, and this should take place alongside identifiable agreed standards. (Clinical Directors)

Senior clinicians in surgery, anaesthesia and medicine need to be involved in the decision to operate on the elderly. Risk assessment must take into account all information strands, including risk factors for acute kidney injury. (Consultants)

An agreed means of assessing frailty in the peri-operative period should be developed and included in risk assessment. (Clinical Directors)

Pain must be assessed and managed as a priority before operation. (Consultants)

All elderly surgical admissions should have a formal nutritional assessment as soon as practicable after their admission so that malnutrition can be identified and managed appropriately. (Trusts, Hospital Nutrition Teams)

***References:***


1. National Confidential Enquiry into Patient Outcome and Death. *Extremes of Age, The 1999 report of the National Confidential Enquiry into Peri-operative Death*. 1999. NCEPOD, London

2. Older P, Smith R et al. Preoperative cardiopulmonary risk assessment by cardiopulmonary exercise testing. *Critical Care and Resuscitation.* 2000; 2(3), 198 - 208

3. Smith TB, Purkayastha S & Paraskevas P. Cardiopulmonary exercise testing as a risk assessment method in non-cardiopulmonary surgery: a systematic review. *Anaesthesia.* 2009; 64(8), 883 - 893

4. Snowden CP, Prentis JM et al. Submaximal cardiopulmonary exercise testing predicts complications and hospital length of stay in patients undergoing major elective surgery. *Annals of Surgery*. 2010; 251(3), 535 - 541

5. Struthers R, Erasmus P et al. Assessing fitness for surgery: a comparison of questionnaire, incremental shuttle walk and cardiopulmonary exercise testing in general surgical patients. *British Journal of Anaesthesia*. 2008; 101(6), 774 - 780

6. Donati M, Ruzzi E et al. A new and feasible model for predicting operative risk. *British Journal of Anaesthesia.* 2004; 93, 393 - 9,

7. Markus PM, Martell J et al. Predicting post operative mortality by clinical assessment. *British Journal of Surgery.* 2005; 92(1), 101 - 106

8. Smith TB, Stonell C et al. Cardioplulmonary exercise testing as a risk assessment method in non cardiopulmonary surgery: a systematic review. *Anaesthesia.* 2009; 64(8), 883 - 893

9. Hightower CE, Riedel BJ et al. A pilot study evaluating predictors of post operative outcomes after major abdominal surgery: physiological capacity compared with ASA physical status classification system. *British Journal of Anaesthesia.* 2010; 104, 465 - 471

10. Tran Ba Loc P, du Montcel ST et al. Elderly POSSUM, a dedicated score for prediction of mortality after major colorectal surgery in older patients. *British Journal of Surgery.* 2010; 97, 396 - 403

11. Department of Health. *The National Service Framework for older people*. 2001. Crown Copyright

12. Royal College of Physicians. *Generic medical record-keeping standards*. 2007. Royal College of Physicians

13. Taylor A. *Nutritional care of older people (skills for caring)*. 2008. M&K Update Ltd

14. British Association of Parenteral and Enteric Nutrition. *Organisation of food and nutritional support in hospitals*. 2007. BAPEN

15. Bradley L & Rees C. Reducing nutritional risk in hospital: the red tray. *Nursing Standard*. 2003; 17(26), 33 - 37

16. Department of Health. *Care homes for older people: national minimum standards and the Care Home Regulations: third edition (revised)*. 2003. Crown Copyright.

17. National Institute for Health and Clinical Excellence. *The management of pressure ulcers in primary and secondary care. A clinical practice guideline*. 2005. Royal College of Nursing and National Institute for Health and Clinical Excellence

18. National Confidential Enquiry into Patient Outcome and Death. *Acute Kidney injury: Adding insult to injury.* 2009. NCEPOD, London

19. Royal College of Physicians, British Geriatric Society & British Pain Society. *National Guideline –the assessment of pain in older people*. 2007. Royal College of Physicians

20. Aubrun F. Management of post operative analgesia in elderly patients. *Regional Anaesthesia and Pain Medicine.* 2005; 30, 363 - 79

21. The Patients Association. *Pain in older people – a hidden problem.* 2007. The Patients Association

22. International Association for Study of Pain. *Facts on Pain in Older Persons.* 2007. www.iasp-pain.org. IASP

23. University of Nottingham & the British Pain Society. *Pain in Older People-Reflections from an older person's perspective.* 2008. Help the Aged.

24. Hadjistavropoulos T, Herr K. An interdisciplinary consensus statement on the assessment of pain in older persons. *Clinical Journal of Pain*. 2007; 23, S1 - 43

25. Royal College of Surgeons England and College of Anaesthetists. Working Party of the Commission on Prevision of Surgical Services. Pain after Surgery. 1990.

# 5 – Intra-operative care

Just over half (585/1085) of the operations were performed by consultant surgeons (Figure 5.1), and consultant anaesthetists were present at the start of the operation in 610/931 cases (not answered in 26). Simlarly consultant anaesthetists also delivered most of the anaesthetics (631/950); this was not answered in 7 cases.

**Table 5.1 Appropriateness of the grade and experience of the most senior surgeon in theatre at the time of operation – Advisors' opinion**

| Grade and experience of surgeon appropriate | n | % |
|---|---|---|
| Yes | 642 | 94.8 |
| No | 35 | 5.2 |
| **Subtotal** | **677** | |
| Unable to answer | 133 | |
| Not answered | 10 | |
| **Total** | **820** | |

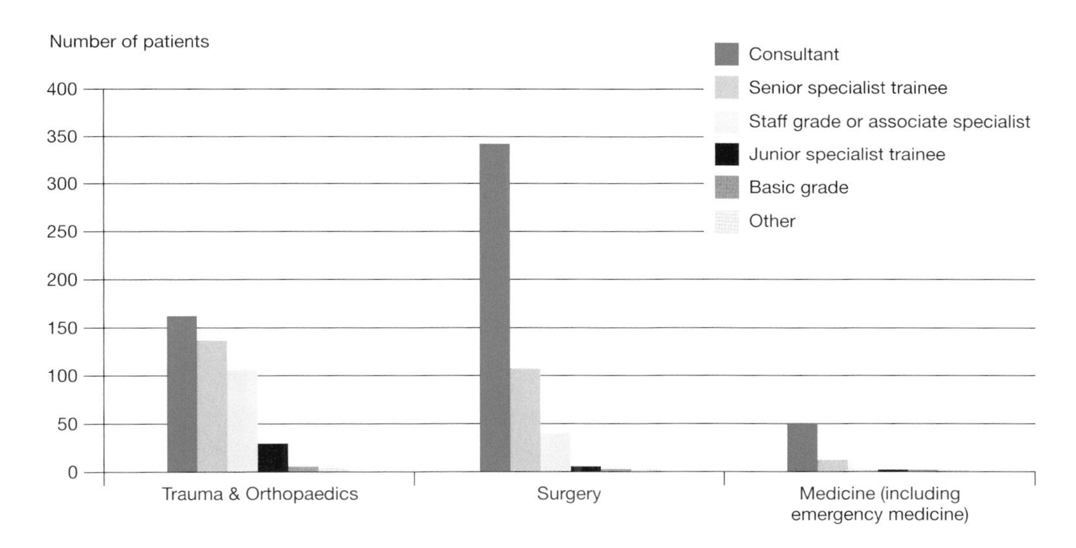


**Figure 5.1. Grade of the most senior operating surgeon by the specialty of clinician proposing the operation**

**Table 5.2 Appropriateness of the specialty of the most senior surgeon in theatre at the time of operation – Advisors' opinion**

| Specialty of surgeon appropriate | n | % |
|---|---|---|
| Yes | 675 | 98.4 |
| No | 11 | 1.6 |
| **Subtotal** | **686** | |
| Unable to answer | 115 | |
| Not answered | 19 | |
| **Total** | **820** | |

In the majority of cases the grade and specialty of the most senior operating surgeon was judged to be appropriate by the Advisors, (Table 5.1 and Table 5.2)

## Surgical supervision

In those cases where the operating surgeon was not a consultant (500/1120) the level of supervision was as shown in Figure 5.2. In only 20.9% (97/464) of cases was the consultant scrubbed in theatre with the trainee or staff grade or associate specialist (SAS). In 30.6% (142/464) the consultant was not in the theatre suite, and in 36.9% (171/464) they were not present in the hospital at the time of surgery. In 54 cases an 'other' answer was selected and in 36 cases the level of supervision was not provided. Of the 142 cases where the consultant was not in the theatre suite, 5 were for more minor procedures; whilst of the 171 operations where the consultant was not present in the hospital 15 were for more minor surgery.

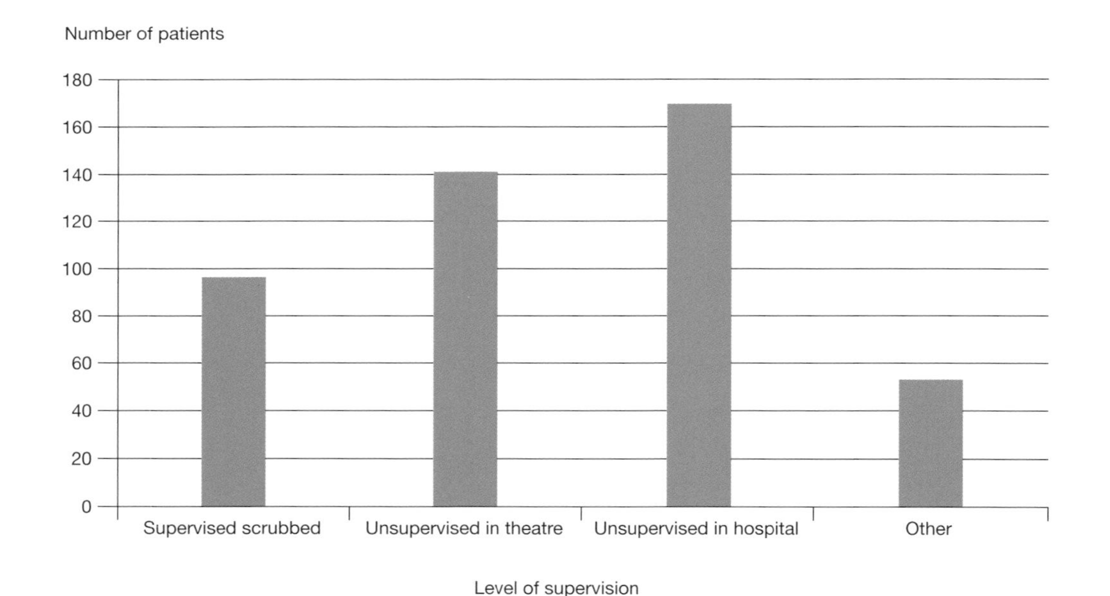


**Figure 5.2. What level of supervision did the primary operator have if they were not a consultant?**

Advisors were asked to assess whether the level of supervision was appropriate given the seniority of trainee, and the complexity of the procedure (Table 5.3).

**Table 5.3 Adequate supervision if the surgeon was not a consultant – Advisors' opinion**

| Level of supervision adequate - surgeon | n | % |
|---|---|---|
| Yes | 126 | 81.8 |
| No | 28 | 18.2 |
| **Subtotal** | **154** | |
| Unable to answer | 130 | |
| Not answered | 44 | |
| **Total** | **328** | |

In the majority of cases where they had sufficient information to make a judgement, Advisors were of the opinion that the level of supervision was adequate. However in 28/154 cases they considered it to be inadequate, and in 130 cases they were unable to answer this question from the information provided. Of the 729 cases where a surgical questionnaire and case notes were returned, 382 cases were operated on by a consultant, and in 19 cases there no answer as to grade of clinician operating.

Further to this, more trauma and orthopaedic (T&O) operations were undertaken by senior trainees and SAS grade doctors, than was the case in general surgery. This will be discussed further in the section on fractured neck of femur.

The following case study presents an example of lack of consultant input and supervision.

**Case study 12**

A patient was admitted with abdominal pain and assessed in the Emergency Department by a junior surgical registrar. A clinical diagnosis of peritonitis was reached. No CT scan was performed and only a full blood count and urea and electrolytes were undertaken. There was no consultant input, and no prophylactic antibiotics were administered. The registrar operated without supervision and discovered acute pancreatitis, and closed the abdomen. The patient was returned to the surgical ward, but after 6 hours the critical care outreach team were called, and the patient was admitted to the Intensive Care Unit and died shortly afterwards of septicaemia.

*Advisors considered that there had been undue haste in proceeding to theatre. More detailed pre-operative investigation and consultant input might have avoided unnecessary surgery.*

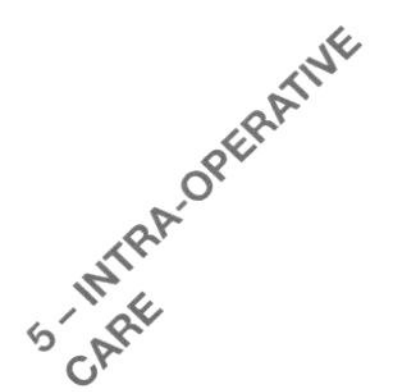


## Junior doctors seeking advice from consultants

**Table 5.4 Evidence that juniors did not seek appropriate consultant advice when necessary – Advisors' opinion**

| Seek appropriate consultant advice | n | % |
|---|---|---|
| Yes | 150 | 19.9 |
| No | 603 | 80.1 |
| **Subtotal** | **753** | |
| Unable to answer | 58 | |
| Not answered | 9 | |
| **Total** | **820** | |

In almost 1 in 5 cases, Advisors found evidence in the notes, which led them to believe that junior doctors had failed to seek appropriate advice from a consultant (Table 5.4). Although the reasons for this may be multi-factorial, it meant that sick and elderly patients were often denied the benefit of input from experienced clinicians at the appropriate time.

**Case study 13**

A patient suffered a post operative upper gastrointestinal bleed from a duodenal ulcer. This was injected by a consultant, and it was clearly documented in the notes that if re-bleed occurred the patient would need open surgery. Despite this when a re-bleed did occur, the junior registrar did not seek consultant advice. Eventually after prolonged attempts at conservative management with fluid resuscitation the patient arrested. It was not clear why the registrar had not followed the management plan and contacted the consultant.

*Advisors noted the lack of communication both in acting on the instructions stated and in seeking advice.*

## Anaesthesia

Anaesthesia was provided by a consultant in 631/950 cases (7 not answered), accompanied by a senior trainee or SAS in 65 cases. Twenty of the 579 patients admitted with an ASA score of 3, 4 and 5 were anaesthetised by a junior or basic grade trainee, and 70/235 ASA 4 patients and 7/30 ASA 5 patients did not have their anaesthetic performed by a consultant. However these latter patients were generally cared for by a senior trainee or SAS grade anaesthetist (Figure 5.3).

As in 1999 the sickest patients were not universally cared for by the most senior anaesthetist.

Advisors were asked whether the grade and experience of the most senior anaesthetist was appropriate (Table 5.5). This was thought to be appropriate in 534/567 cases, but was not in 33/567 cases. Advisors were unable to answer this or did not answer this in 253 cases, probably because the grade of the anaesthetist was impossible to ascertain from notes retrospectively. It is a recommendation of the Royal College of Anaesthetists that the grade of anaesthetist (and in the case of a trainee the grade of the supervising anaesthetist) be noted on the anaesthetic record.[1]

**Table 5.5 Appropriateness of the grade and experience of the most senior anaesthetist for the anaesthetic care of the patient – Advisors' opinion**

| Senior anaesthetist appropriate to the care of the patient | n | % |
|---|---|---|
| Yes | 534 | 94.2 |
| No | 33 | 5.8 |
| **Subtotal** | **567** | |
| Unable to answer | 216 | |
| Not answered | 37 | |
| **Total** | **820** | |

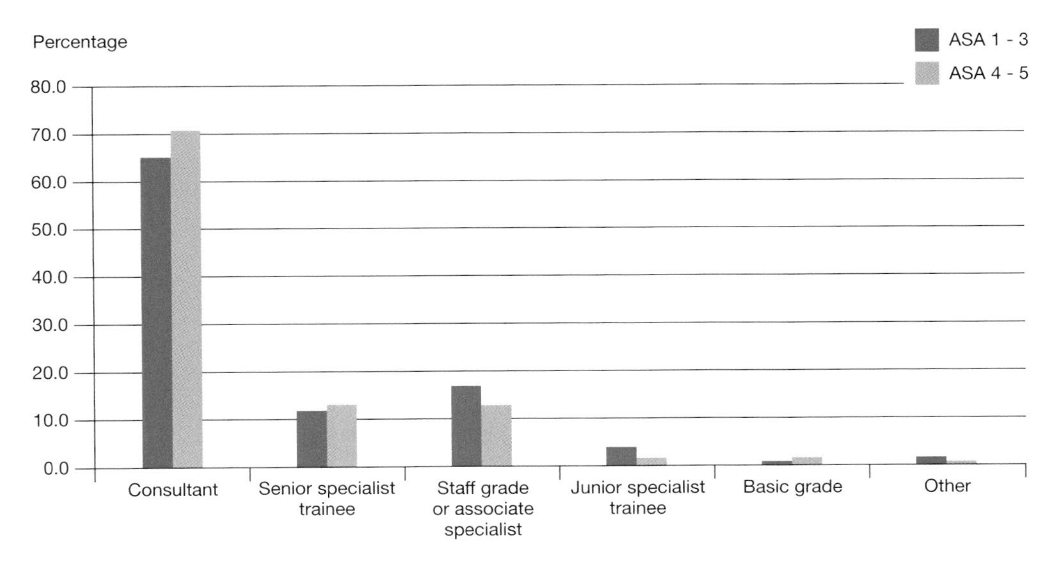


**Figure 5.3. Grade of anaesthetist providing the anaesthetic by ASA prior to surgery**

In the majority of cases, Advisors were of the opinion that the grade and experience of the anaesthetists was appropriate to the care required by the patient.

## Type of anaesthetic

380/946 underwent general anaesthetic alone, 354/946 regional or neuraxial block with GA or sedation and 128/946 underwent unsupplemented spinal anaesthesia, with or without a nerve block. The remaining 84 patients received multiple methods of anaesthesia. In 11 cases the type of anaesthesic could not be determined.

## Anaesthetic supervision

In 319 cases the anaesthetic was not provided by a consultant. Whilst in many cases (139/263) the consultant was present in the theatre suite, in about half (119/263) the supervising consultant was either elsewhere in the hospital, or only available by telephone. In 5 cases the clinician completing the questionnaire gave an alternative answer, and further information was not provided in 56 cases.

**Table 5.6 Adequate supervision if the anaesthetist was not a consultant – Advisors' opinion**

| Level of supervision appropriate – anaesthetist | n | % |
|---|---|---|
| Yes | 81 | 82.7 |
| No | 17 | 17.3 |
| **Subtotal** | **98** | |
| Unable to answer | 63 | |
| Not answered | 27 | |
| **Total** | **188** | |

Of the 588 cases where an anaesthetic questionnaire and case notes were returned, 188 cases were not anaesthetised by a consultant. In most cases where an anaesthetic was administered by a trainee Advisors were of the opinion that the level of supervision was appropriate although in 17 where they were able to make a determination, they considered the level of supervision was inappropriate. 395 were anaesthetised by a consultant; in 5 cases the grade of anaesthetist providing the anaesthetic was not given (Table 5.6).

### Anaesthetic monitoring

Table 5.7 demonstrates the relative frequency of monitoring undertaken in this group of patients, over and above the basic minimum levels of mandatory monitoring for any patient undergoing surgery. In 103 cases this question was not answered.

**Table 5.7 Above minimum levels of anaesthetic monitoring**

| Anaesthetic monitoring | n* |
|---|---|
| Temperature | 394 |
| Arterial BP | 366 |
| Blood gases | 265 |
| CVP | 254 |
| Other near patient testing | 168 |
| Cardiac output | 49 |
| Depth of anaesthesia | 39 |
| None additional | 293 |

**Answers may be multiple*

In the majority of cases, Advisors were of the opinion that the level of physiological monitoring was appropriate (Table 5.8). However there were a number of concerns about the recording of monitoring in the case notes, and in particular the monitoring of temperature, which is of importance in elderly patients.

**Table 5.8 – Adequacy of the physiological monitoring – Advisors' opinion**

| Adequate physiological monitoring | n | % |
|---|---|---|
| Yes | 607 | 89.5 |
| No | 71 | 10.5 |
| **Subtotal** | **678** | |
| Unable to answer | 117 | |
| Not answered | 25 | |
| **Total** | **820** | |

### Temperature management

Peri-operative hypothermia is common in both young and old patients undergoing a surgical procedure.[2,3,4] However the course of this is likely to be longer and more pronounced in the elderly who have reduced muscle mass and a compromised ability to regain effective thermoregulatory control. Adverse consequences of peri-operative hypothermia include cardiac ischaemia and arrhythmias, increased blood loss, wound infection, decreased drug metabolism and increased post operative stay.

As Table 5.9 indicates, whilst it was clear from the case notes that 81% of patients had temperature monitoring in the post operative period, only half of the case notes contained evidence of monitoring in the immediate pre-operative period and during surgery. It was also notable that during all phases of the peri-operative period, the use of temperature monitoring could not be assessed in a substantial number of cases. Advisors were surprised to note that not all peri-operative and anaesthetic monitoring charts had a section requiring the recording of temperature.

Table 5.9 Peri-operative temperature monitoring – Advisor assessment from case notes

| Temperature measured | | Yes | | No | Subtotal | Unable to answer/ not answered | Total |
|---|---|---|---|---|---|---|---|
| | n | % | n | % | n | n | n |
| Immediately pre-operatively | 293 | 54.4 | 246 | 45.6 | **539** | 281 | **820** |
| Intra-operatively | 313 | 49.7 | 317 | 50.3 | **630** | 190 | **820** |
| Post operatively | 483 | 80.9 | 114 | 19.1 | **597** | 223 | **820** |

## Warming devices

The recorded use of warming devices was also poor (Table 5.10).

Table 5.10 Use of warming devices – Advisor assessment from the case notes

| Warming devices used | | Yes | | No | Subtotal | Unable to answer/ not answered | Total |
|---|---|---|---|---|---|---|---|
| | n | % | n | % | n | n | n |
| Warmed fluids | 248 | 55.4 | 200 | 44.6 | **448** | 372 | **820** |
| Forced air warming devices | 313 | 67.3 | 152 | 32.7 | **465** | 355 | **820** |
| Low flow anaesthesia | 136 | 39.8 | 206 | 60.2 | **342** | 478 | **820** |

The recorded use of warming techniques during surgery was incomplete ranging from forced air devices in 67% of patients, to warmed fluids in 55%, and apparently low flow anaesthesia in under 40%.

In the post anaesthesia care unit there was even less evidence of active warming being undertaken (Table 5.11), with around 67% receiving temperature measurement, 20% receiving warmed fluids and 25% forced air warming.

It is not possible to determine from these data, whether the management of temperature was deficient, or whether this is simply a reflection of poor record keeping. Whatever it adds further support to the need for greater standardisation of both the content and layout of peri-operative and intra-operative records.

**Table 5.11 Documented evidence of temperature maintenance in the recovery unit/post anaesthesia care unit (PACU)**

| Temperature maintenance in recovery/ PACU | Yes | | No | | Subtotal | Unable to answer/ not answered | Total |
|---|---|---|---|---|---|---|---|
| | n | % | n | % | n | n | n |
| Temperature measurement | 367 | 67.1 | 180 | 32.9 | **547** | 273 | **820** |
| Warmed fluids | 76 | 20.7 | 292 | 79.3 | **368** | 452 | **820** |
| Forced air warming | 88 | 25.1 | 263 | 74.9 | **351** | 469 | **820** |

The following case study demonstrates a lack of post operative temperature maintenance

**Case study 14**

At the start of an elective anterior resection, a patient was noted to have a temperature of 35.2°C and became more hypothermic at 34.8°C over the two hour procedure. On return to the surgical ward the patient was noted to be shivering and had a temperature of 35.5°C. The temperature had been monitored in theatre, and warmed fluids and a forced air warming device had been used. However these were not continued in recovery, and no temperature monitoring was undertaken prior to surgery or in recovery. The patient remained hypothermic for 7 hours in the post operative period, and was managed with warmed fluids and a space blanket. The patient eventually succumbed to peritonitis secondary to ischaemic bowel.

*Advisors were of the view that inadequate attention had been paid to the hypothermia and that no effective attempts had been made to correct this throughout the post operative period.*

## Anaesthetic complications

**Table 5.12 Anaesthetic related complication – Advisors' opinion**

| Anaesthetic complications | n | % |
|---|---|---|
| Yes | 108 | 15.1 |
| No | 609 | 84.9 |
| **Subtotal** | **717** | |
| Unable to answer | 55 | |
| Not answered | 48 | |
| **Total** | **820** | |

Complications related to the anaesthetic occurred in 15.1% (108/717) of cases (Table 5.12), and where it could be determined the outcome was adversely affected in 56/84 cases. Advisors were unable to assess this in 22 cases and did not answer in 2.

## Peri-operative hypotension

There is no universal definition of peri-operative hypotension in terms of level (systolic), duration, or means of measurement. Following discussion with the Expert Group, it was decided that 90mmHg was a level below which there would be definite concern amongst clinicians in the elderly population under review, and at which active management is likely to be required.

Thus 438/937 (46.7%) patients had episodes of hypotension (unknown in 12 cases and not answered in 20). Whilst reviews of anaesthesia for the elderly suggest keeping blood pressure within 20% to 30% of pre-anaesthetic levels, it is important to note that there is no absolute level which prevents post operative complications. However, peri-operative hypotension has certainly been linked with myocardial ischaemia, cerebro-vascular events and post operative confusion.

Problems may also be encountered in the elderly with hypertension, as they may demonstrate marked lability of blood pressure, even when on a stable regimen of medication pre-operatively.

Hypotension may be an indicator of reduced cardiac output, measurement of which may pose challenges within a theatre setting. Nevertheless real time non invasive cardiac output measurement is increasingly available and used for high risk patients e.g. in the context of vascular surgery. Where appropriate these same "gold standards" should be applied to elderly sick laparotomy or revision arthroplasty patients. Measurements can then be used to guide judicious use of fluids, inotropes and vasoconstrictors.

Even without the availability of more sophisticated monitoring, strict attention to blood pressure control alongside other parameters is good practice particularly in this type of patient, and it is probable that a conscious decision to maintain blood pressure within certain limits will improve outcome.

The following case study illustrates problems with peri-operative hypotension.

**Case study 15**

A patient with a moderate degree of scoliosis presented with a fractured neck of femur. Pre-operative blood pressure was 142/97 and was noted to be 120/80 prior to a spinal anaesthetic being administered. This was performed by a junior anaesthetist and was noted to be difficult, with 5 attempts before success. The patient had a period during which systolic blood pressure was noted to be < 80mmHg, the lowest blood pressure being 50mmHg. Treatment included 1.5 litres of fluid and intravenous metaraminol. The patient appeared to have had continued hypotension in the recovery room and a post operative myocardial infarction resulted in death.

*Advisors commented that the dose of local anaesthetic used for the spinal block was relatively large and that more aggressive management of blood pressure may have improved outcome. Senior input should also have been sought.*

## Cardio-pulmonary instability

There were substantial problems with intra-operative blood pressure control in 438/937 cases, suspected cardiac ischaemia in 49/928 cases, rhythm problems in 136/914, and problems maintaining oxygenation in 60/925 (Table 5.13).

Cardiovascular complications are known to be particularly common in the elderly peri-operative population and contribute significantly to morbidity and mortality.[5] These are a result of reduced physiological reserve, pre-existing cardiac and vascular disease, and the additional effects of the acute surgical illness (such as sepsis and dehydration).

**Table 5.13 Intra-operative problems with blood pressure, cardiac ischaemia, heart rate or rhythm or maintaining oxygenation**

| Intra operative problems | Yes | | No | | Unknown | | Subtotal | Not answered | Total |
|---|---|---|---|---|---|---|---|---|---|
| | n | % | n | % | n | % | n | n | n |
| Blood pressure instability (Systolic blood pressure (SABP) <90mmHg) | 438 | 46.7 | 487 | 52 | 12 | 1.3 | **937** | 20 | **957** |
| Suspected cardiac ischaemia | 49 | 5.3 | 794 | 85.6 | 85 | 9.2 | **928** | 29 | **957** |
| Heart rate or rhythm | 136 | 14.9 | 754 | 82.5 | 24 | 2.6 | **914** | 43 | **957** |
| Maintaining oxygenation | 60 | 6.5 | 858 | 92.8 | 7 | <1 | **925** | 32 | **957** |

## Key findings

Consultant involvement in care was high in this group of patients and in most cases the experience of both the surgeon and anaesthetist was judged to be appropriate to the care needs of the patient.

There was frequently a lack of evidence of the monitoring of temperature, and recording of therapeutic interventions to prevent hypothermia within this sample.

Peri-operative hypotension was a common event in this population (438/937), and is likely to have contributed to poor outcome.

## Recommendations

Temperature monitoring and management of hypothermia should be recorded in a nationally standardised anaesthetic record. This is particularly important in elderly patients. (Clinical Directors)

There should be clear strategies for the management of intra-operative low blood pressure in the elderly to avoid cardiac and renal complications. Non invasive measurement of cardiac output facilitates this during major surgery in the elderly. (Clinical Directors)

### *References*

1. Royal College of Anaesthetists and Association of Anaesthetists of Great Britain and Ireland. *Good Practice. A guide for departments of anaesthesia, critical care and pain management.* Third edition, 2006. Royal College of Anaesthetists and Association of Anaesthetists of Great Britain and Ireland

2. Sessler DI. Mile peri-operative hypothermia. *New England Medical Journal*. 1997; 336, 1730 - 1737

3. El-Gamal N, El-Kassabany N et al. Age-related thermoregulatory differences in a warm operating room environment (approximately 26 degrees C). *Anaesthesia Analgesia.* 2000; 90(3), 694 - 698

4. National Institute for Health and Clinical Excellence. *The management of inadvertent perioperative hypothermia in adults.* 2008. NICE

5. Bijker Jb, van Klei WA et al. Intraoperative hypotension and 1-year mortality after Noncardiac surgery. *Anaesthesiology.* 2009; 111(6), 1217 - 1226

# 6 – Post operative care

## Admission to intensive care

The 1999 NCEPOD report recommended that:
*"If a decision is made to operate then that must include a decision to provide appropriate post operative care that may include HDU/ICU support. It is accepted that intra-operative findings e.g. disseminated malignancy may subsequently influence post operative management".*[1]

Nevertheless that report found that in a population of over 90's undergoing surgery just 6% of patients received care in an Intensive Care Unit (ICU) and 4% in a High Dependency Unit (HDU) immediately after leaving theatre/ recovery.

In the 10 years following this, ICU and HDU capacity in the UK has increased substantially.[2,3] Similarly there has been a marked coincident increase in the elderly population, and attitudes to care provision may also have changed. In this study we note that 216/1073 received level 2 or 3 care immediately after leaving theatre (Table 6.1), and a further 106 patients went on to receive this after leaving the theatre recovery suite (Table 6.2). Thus a total of 322 patients (about a third of our population) received level 2 or 3 care in the early post operative period.

Of the 710 patients admitted to recovery, most (543/659) were then transferred to a specialist or general ward area (Table 6.2). It may be that some of the specialised ward areas provided enhanced care, but there was no information for this.

**Table 6.1 Location where the patient was admitted immediately after leaving the theatre/operating area**

| Area of care following surgery | n | % |
|---|---|---|
| Recovery suite | 710 | 66.2 |
| Level 3 | 182 | 17.0 |
| Level 2 | 34 | 3.2 |
| Specialist ward | 63 | 5.9 |
| General ward | 50 | 4.7 |
| Other | 12 | 1.1 |
| Mortuary | 22 | 2.1 |
| **Subtotal** | **1073** | |
| Not answered | 47 | |
| **Total** | **1120** | |

**Table 6.2 Location where the patient was admitted following recovery**

| Area of care following recovery | n | % |
|---|---|---|
| Level 3 | 46 | 7.0 |
| Level 2 | 60 | 9.1 |
| Specialist ward | 351 | 53.3 |
| General ward | 192 | 29.1 |
| Other | 10 | 1.5 |
| **Subtotal** | **659** | |
| Not answered | 42 | |
| Died in theatre | 9 | |
| **Total** | **710** | |

Anaesthetists completing the questionnaire were asked if they were aware whether patients received extended recovery, and in 199/854 cases this had occurred (Table 6.3). Some of these may have ultimately been admitted to level 2 or 3 care.

**Table 6.3 Receipt of extended recovery**

| Extended recovery | n | % |
|---|---|---|
| Yes | 199 | 23.3 |
| No | 623 | 73.0 |
| Unknown | 32 | 3.7 |
| **Subtotal** | **854** | |
| Not answered | 103 | |
| **Total** | **957** | |

In this study most patients received the level of care planned for them post operatively, for example 292/790 cases were planned to have level 2 or 3 care and 287/790 received it (Table 6.4).

Despite these findings and given the high burden of comorbidity in this population it may be surprising that a greater number of patients did not have enhanced care planned for them. Advisors indicated that there may have often been low expectations, and that this affected judgements about what level of care was both planned and received. Denying access to services based on age alone is unacceptable[6,7] and decisions must be made on the basis of health needs and the possibility of benefiting from this care. This in turn is a matter for careful pre-operative evaluation and planning as discussed in chapter 3.

**Table 6.4 Planned level of care by actual level of care**

| | | Actual level of care (n) | | | | | | |
|---|---|---|---|---|---|---|---|---|
| **Level of care** | | **Level 1** | **Level 2** | **Level 3** | **Unknown** | **Subtotal** | **Not answered** | **Total** |
| **Planned level of care (n)** | **Level 1** | 451 | 3 | 0 | 13 | **467** | 8 | **475** |
| | **Level 2** | 6 | 114 | 8 | 2 | **130** | 5 | **135** |
| | **Level 3** | 1 | 0 | 161 | 0 | **162** | 9 | **171** |
| | **Unknown** | 7 | 1 | 0 | 23 | **31** | 3 | **34** |
| | **Subtotal** | **465** | **118** | **169** | **38** | **790** | **25** | **815** |
| | **Not answered** | 7 | 3 | 5 | 0 | **15** | 127 | **142** |
| | **Total** | **472** | **121** | **174** | **38** | **805** | **152** | **957** |

The most recent Intensive Care National Audit and Research Network (ICNARC) data set suggests that nationally about 14% of ICU admissions were in the over 80 age group.[4] However it is clear that this varies across the world with over 65s occupying up to 51% of ICU beds in a recent literature review of outcome in the elderly intensive care patients.[5]

Advisors were asked whether they thought that patients who did not go to critical care had received the most appropriate care post operatively. In 67/508 cases where an opinion was recorded, the Advisors indicated patients did not go to the most appropriate ward (Table 6.5).

**Table 6.5 Appropriateness of the post operative ward if the patient did not receive level 2 or 3 care – Advisors' opinion**

| Appropriate post operative ward care | n | % |
|---|---|---|
| Yes | 441 | 87.0 |
| No | 67 | 13.2 |
| **Subtotal** | **508** | |
| Unable to answer | 76 | |
| Not applicable/ answered | 236 | |
| **Total** | **820** | |

The following case study presents an example of poor level 2 care planning.

**Case study 16**

A patient underwent planned revision knee surgery, having been hospitalised for several months with immobility. Associated problems included atrial fibrillation, hypertension and a previous cerebrovascular accident. Blood loss was moderate and the patient was noted to have a post operative haemoglobin of 8g/dl. Analgesia consisted of a nerve block and systemic opioids. Within 12 hours of surgery the patient had developed reduced oxygen saturation and hypotension and was treated with additional fluids and oxygen. The patient subsequently had a post operative myocardial infarction, developed pulmonary oedema and a chest infection. Only on day 21 when the condition again deteriorated was a higher level of care contemplated.

*Advisors felt it was unsatisfactory that level 2 care had not been planned for this patient pre-operatively.*

Several studies have pointed to the fact that it is not age alone which determines outcome in the elderly intensive care patient. In a study of 255 octogenarians receiving intensive care following major bowel surgery[8], the most important predictor of outcome was the requirement for vaso-active drugs. Age alone was not a good predictive factor, and there was a marked difference in mortality between elective and emergency surgery (21% mortality in elective cases vs. 42% in emergencies). In a further study, age only correlated with survival when related to the use of invasive ventilation. If patients did not require ventilation there was no effect of age on ICU survival.[9] It is also important to note that research on functional status in the elderly survivors of intensive care tends to indicate that there is less disruption to life than may be seen in the younger patient[10] which may indicate that despite the challenges of comorbidity, disability and frailty, the elderly are often easier to return to their pre-operative status and quality of life.

Advisors recorded that there were a relatively large (72/793) number of unforeseen admissions to critical care, (unable to answer in 8 cases and did not answer in 19). On occasion this may have been as a result of unexpected surgical findings or complications. However, with careful diagnostic workup and discussion the majority of these should have been avoidable. The implications of unanticipated admission are substantial and are linked to poor outcome.[11] Unanticipated admissions demonstrate a failure of risk assessment and have critical day to day effects on resource planning within critical care units.

Advisors were asked about their views on where the elderly should best be cared for after surgery, as there is unlikely to be a further expansion in critical care provision in the near future. Suggested models included extended recovery, or a "Post Anaesthesia Care unit" (PACU) for 12-24 hours post operatively for more straightforward procedures. As an alternative, designated peri-operative "bays" in wards supported by input from Medicine for the Care of Older People (MCOP) clinicians may be effective.

Though this study indicated that a relatively large number of sick post operative elderly patients now receive level 2 and 3 care, there may still be a shortfall.

Advisors again commented that there was a low expectation for these patients and that it may well have been extreme old age and urgency of surgery that affected judgement as to location of care. In some cases the fact that surgery was relatively minor may have also affected decision making.

## Did the right patients go to ICU?

Planned level of care was further explored against health status using the ASA score. Of those patients where level 2 care was planned post operatively, 14/99 were ASA 2, 50/99 ASA 3, 30/99 ASA 4 and 5/99 ASA 5 (in 3 cases not answered). Of those where there was a plan to receive level 3 care post operatively 13/131 were ASA 2, 46/131 were ASA 3, 55/131 ASA 4, and 17/131 ASA 5 (again in 3 cases this was not answered). Predictably it was generally the sickest patients that went to HDU/ICU.[12]

Generally whilst patients requiring surgery for fractured neck of femur were less sick based on ASA grade than those undergoing abdominal surgery, far fewer had level 2 or 3 care planned (32/251 NOF cases, as opposed to 106/157 acute abdomen). This is not surprising given the underlying diagnosis in the patients undergoing emergency abdominal surgery, the length of procedure and greater blood and fluid losses. Nevertheless the fractured neck of femur group was not homogeneous, with some requiring more complex surgery and many having serious concurrent illness associated with their injury. Management of this on a busy post operative orthopaedic ward may be far from optimal.

## Post operative acute kidney injury (AKI)

Where AKI developed post admission (n=248), Advisors were asked when this was first noted. In 63% of patients (151/238) AKI was first noted post operatively (Table 6.6).

**Table 6.6 First identification of AKI – Advisors' opinion**

| When AKI was noted | n | % |
|---|---|---|
| Pre-operatively | 87 | 36.6 |
| Post operatively | 151 | 63.4 |
| **Subtotal** | **238** | |
| Unable to answer | 8 | |
| Not answered/not applicable | 2 | |
| **Total** | **248** | |

Where AKI developed post operatively it was the Advisors' opinion that this was due to surgical complications in 46 patients. Even with the best surgical technique complications can occur, thus AKI in this group was not necessarily a reflection of poor practice; indeed our Advisors found only one case of AKI being related to poor surgical technique. However, in their opinion, 46 patients received poor pre/intra-operative care and 39 poor post operative care resulting in AKI. In a further 22 it was the result of poor pre-operative resuscitation and in 7 it at least in part arose due to delays in surgery (Table 6.7).

Table 6.7 Reasons for post operative AKI – Advisors' opinion

| Reasons for post operative AKI | n* |
|---|---|
| Complications of surgery | 46 |
| Poor post operative management | 39 |
| Poor intra-operative management of fluids/cardiovascular status | 24 |
| Unsatisfactory pre-operative resuscitation | 22 |
| Timeliness of surgery | 7 |
| Poor surgical technique | 1 |
| Other | 42 |
| Unable to answer | 16 |

*answers may be multiple*

As previously mentioned elderly surgical patients are at an inherent risk of AKI and a lack of attention to supportive renal care in the peri-operative period is a regrettable oversight.[13] For instance, despite the majority of patients having adequate checks on their urea and electrolytes (553), only 371/912 patients had hourly urine output measured (45 not answered). Anaesthetists completing the questionnaire also indicated that 11.6% of patients (99/850) had inadequate urine output during the intra-operative period (for 464/850, 54.6% of patients it was impossible for the responding clinicians to tell, and was not answered by an additional 107 clinicians). Intra-operatively 36.6% (337/920) of patients did not have fluid input/output measured (Table 6.8), with 46.7% (438/937) having labile intra-operative blood pressure, (unknown in 37 cases). Additionally, the quality of the fluid balance charts received was deemed poor or unacceptable by Advisors in 116 cases, good in 153 cases, satisfactory in 355.

Table 6.8 Aspects of intra-operative fluid management documented

| Intra-operative fluid documentation | n | % |
|---|---|---|
| Fluid input | 581 | 63.2 |
| Fluid input and urine output | 337 | 36.6 |
| Urine output | 2 | 0.3 |
| **Subtotal** | **920** | |
| Not answered | 37 | |
| **Total** | **957** | |

Fortunately the majority of patients with AKI were in Stage 1 (186/277) when it was diagnosed (Table 6.9), the implication being that it was either detected early or had not progressed. However it is of concern, that our Advisors considered that 33 patients had an unacceptable delay in the recognition of their AKI with eight patients being in AKI for greater than 3 or more days before it was diagnosed.

Table 6.9 Stage of AKI the patient was in when it was first recognised – Advisors' opinion

| Stage AKI when detected | n | % |
|---|---|---|
| Stage 1 | 186 | 67.1 |
| Stage 2 | 70 | 25.3 |
| Stage 3 | 21 | 7.6 |
| **Subtotal** | **277** | |
| Unable to answer | 58 | |
| Not answered/NA | 485 | |
| **Total** | **820** | |

AKI may on occasion be an unavoidable complication. However good pre-operative assessment and resuscitation, appropriate intra-operative care (including recording of fluid balance and maintenance of renal perfusion), coupled with ward medical staff being alert to the risk of AKI in the post operative period should significantly reduce morbidity in this group.[13] Principle recommendations from the *Adding Insult to Injury* NCEPOD report can be found in Appendix 1.

## Place of death

**Table 6.10 Place of death**

| Place of death | n | % |
|---|---|---|
| Anaesthetic room | 2 | <1 |
| Theatre | 31 | 2.8 |
| Level 3 | 203 | 18.7 |
| Level 2 | 49 | 4.5 |
| Recovery room | 16 | 1.5 |
| Specialist ward | 441 | 40.5 |
| General ward | 336 | 30.9 |
| Other | 10 | <1 |
| **Subtotal** | **1088** | |
| Not answered | 32 | |
| **Total** | **1120** | |

As Table 6.10 demonstrates 252/1088 cases died in level 2 or 3 care. ICU survival is more closely linked to the level of support required rather than age. Whilst ASA 4 and 5 patients will nearly always be admitted to this level of care on occasion it may be appropriate to consider end of life care far sooner in the elderly. If possible this should be broached with the patient and carers pre-operatively so that their views may be taken into account before major surgery is performed and particularly if the outcome is predicted to be poor.

49/1088 patients died in the theatre suite (anaesthetic room, operating theatre and recovery). Whilst this is a relatively small number, and probably unavoidable, such deaths are likely to be traumatic for the family, carers and clinicians involved.[14]

In the majority (43/49) of cases we noted that the decision to operate, in those patients who died in theatre, was made (appropriately) by a consultant. In the remaining 5 cases a decision was made by a senior trainee (not answered in 1 case).

Whilst we were concerned that on occasion high dependency and intensive care was not made available, there were several cases where concerns were raised that relatively aggressive treatment was given and that consideration should have been given to what limits on treatment there should be. In the opinion of our Advisors decisions to stop aggressive post operative medical treatment were sometimes made late.

**Case study 17**

A patient who was frail but "well for their age" with no specific co-morbidity noted had an uneventful operation for fractured neck of femur sustained by a fall. 13 days post operatively a chest infection developed, and relatively soon afterwards the patient had a cardiac arrest on the ward. No do not attempt resuscitation discussions had taken place. It was documented that "3 rounds of cardiopulmonary resuscitation" were undertaken before treatment was eventually withdrawn.

*Whilst discussions about what a patient wishes to occur in such circumstances may be difficult to initiate, they should nonetheless be undertaken, and it is the responsibility of attendant clinician to document clearly that they have taken place.*

## Post operative pain management

Advisors were asked whether there was evidence that pain was assessed regularly post operatively (Table 6.11).

**Table 6.11 Evidence that pain was assessed regularly in the post operative period – Advisors' opinion**

| Post operative pain assessment | n | % |
|---|---|---|
| Yes | 477 | 77.9 |
| No | 135 | 22.1 |
| **Subtotal** | **612** | |
| Unable to answer | 181 | |
| Not answered | 27 | |
| **Total** | **820** | |

In 477 patients Advisors were able to find some evidence of regular pain assessment in the notes, but in135 cases this was not recorded, and not answered in 181. In 1999 only 235/944 anaesthetic questionnaires reported that the patient had a pain assessment chart, and in some cases this related only to the time during which the patient was in the recovery area.

When pain assessment tools were used Advisors were also asked to assess from the notes whether these had been modified in the light of sensory impairment. In 112/139 cases where Advisors believed that scoring should have been modified this was done (Table 6.12).

**Table 6.12 Where pain was assessed regularly, efforts were made to modify pain scoring in light of sensory impairment**

| Modified pain scoring | n | % |
|---|---|---|
| Yes | 112 | 80.6 |
| No | 27 | 19.4 |
| **Subtotal** | **139** | |
| Unable to answer | 133 | |
| Not applicable | 169 | |
| Not answered | 36 | |
| **Total** | **477** | |

As previously indicated, a substantial proportion of the population (299/820) had one or more sensory or communication problems and may have benefited from more sophisticated pain assessment tools. Whilst there are various tools which facilitate pain assessment in patients with communication problems, there is a lack of standardisation in this area.

Elderly patients are generally reluctant to report pain and should be specifically asked about it in any assessment. Alternative descriptors are often used, and careful observation as well as verbal history is important, especially in patients with comprehension and communication problems. In order to perform this effectively there needs to be familiarity with the type of behaviour that may indicate pain. Regular carers often have important insights in this type of assessment and should be asked for their input when possible.

Advisors were asked for their opinion on whether adequate analgesia was provided post operatively (Table 6.13).

**Table 6.13 Adequacy of analgesia received post operatively – Advisors' opinion**

| Adequate post operative analgesia | n | % |
|---|---|---|
| Yes | 559 | 92.9 |
| No | 43 | 7.1 |
| **Subtotal** | **602** | |
| Unable to answer | 186 | |
| Not answered | 32 | |
| **Total** | **820** | |

In the majority of patients analgesia provision was thought to be adequate but in 43 patients it was not. In a further 186 cases the advisor was unable to make a judgement on this.

There is evidence that there are particularly likely to be problems with under-treatment in patients with cognitive impairment.[15] There may also be issues of over treatment or inappropriate use of opiates, particularly in patients with communication difficulties. This is illustrated in case study 18.

Analgesia was prescribed regularly post operatively in the vast majority of patients; in a small number (39/653) this was not the case (Table 6.14). Whilst dosing intervals should ideally be individualised according to the patient's condition and needs, generally there is a need for a multi-modal approach which includes some form of regular analgesia. It should be recognised that care needs to be taken when prescribing in terms of route of administration, dose, duration and potential cross reactions with other medication.[15] Particular care should be taken with non steroidal anti-inflammatory agents which may precipitate acute renal failure in the elderly. Doses of opioids generally need to be reduced, but there is marked inter-patient variability so dose titration is required with careful monitoring of sedation. Concerns about use of opioids in those with cognitive impairment are unfounded and studies suggest that appropriate opioid based pain management in the elderly may actually improve cognitive function.[16] Many side effects of opioids are reduced in the elderly, for example post operative nausea and vomiting.

**Table 6.14 Evidence of analgesia being prescribed regularly in the post operative period – Advisors' opinion**

| Regular post operative analgesia | n | % |
|---|---|---|
| Yes | 614 | 94.0 |
| No | 39 | 6.0 |
| **Subtotal** | **653** | |
| Not answered | 16 | |
| Unable to answer | 109 | |
| Not applicable | 42 | |
| **Total** | **820** | |

Anaesthetists completing the questionnaire were asked which types of pain relief were prescribed post operatively. Paracetamol and oral opiates were the most popular choice, with relatively limited use of epidural analgesia and patient controlled analgesia (Table 6.15).

**Table 6.15 Methods of post operative pain relief**

| Pain relief | n* |
|---|---|
| Paracetamol | 633 |
| Oral opioid analgesia | 361 |
| Intravenous or intramuscular bolus opioid | 353 |
| Other | 107 |
| Epidural | 102 |
| Patient controlled analgesia | 87 |
| Non steroidal anti inflammatory (NSAID) | 28 |

*answers may be multiple*

**Case study 18**

A patient was admitted from a nursing home after a fall. There was a known history of dementia and the patient was extremely agitated in the Emergency Department where they received an initial 24mg of morphine. The patient went to theatre less than 24 hours later by which time a further 20mg of morphine and 4mg of diazepam had been given. The consultant anaesthetist commented that the patient was "unrousable" in the anaesthetic room, and was given a spinal anaesthetic for their surgery. No further analgesia appeared to have been given post operatively. Death followed 10 days later from a chest infection.

*Advisors commented that whilst it may have been difficult to assess pain and administer appropriate analgesia in a patient with severe dementia, at the very least simple analgesics should have been administered if necessary using a parenteral route.*

The analgesia received by those patients who underwent emergency abdominal surgery was explored in more detail. A minority (44/186) received epidural analgesia (Table 6.16).

The 1999 report[1] commented upon the fact that there were cases where epidural analgesia combined with general anaesthesia had been in part responsible for intra-operative hypotension, and that careful management was required particularly if hypovolaemia was also present.

**Table 6.16 Methods of post operative pain relief within patients undergoing abdominal surgery**

| Post operative pain relief | n* |
|---|---|
| Paracetamol | 88 |
| IV or IM bolus | 76 |
| Epidural | 44 |
| Patient controlled analgaesia | 36 |
| Oral opiod analgesia | 18 |
| NSAID | 3 |
| Other | 26 |

**answers may be multiple*

Analgesia for major abdominal surgery in the elderly as with any other group, should be planned in advance, and regional block is an effective adjunct to general anaesthesia. However continuous epidural analgesia needs to be managed in an appropriately supervised setting by staff familiar with the management of this form of analgesia and any complications which may ensue.[17] This should be supplemented by input from an acute pain service. In the elderly, epidurals should be managed with careful incremental dosing or preferably by continuous infusion using the lowest possible effective concentration of drugs to minimise complications.

Evidence also exists that Patient Controlled Analgesia (PCA) can be used effectively in the elderly.[18] However adaptations may need to be made in those with reduced hand strength and mobility. Generally opioid use is less than in younger subjects. In the current study only 36/186 patients undergoing abdominal surgery received PCA (Table 6.16).

There is evidence that PCA and epidural analgesia are more effective in the elderly than conventional opioid regimens.[15] Given the anticipated severity of pain associated with abdominal surgery we were surprised to find that so few patients benefited from the use of continuous analgesia techniques. This may reflect an under-estimate of need, a perception that these techniques are particularly high risk, or possibly poor access to the correct post operative facilities.

**Case study 19**

A patient with dementia and poor nutrition presented with fractured NOF, and a past history of myocardial infarction, multiple myeloma and chronic kidney disease. Surgery was expedited in a timely fashion, but the patient became drowsy 24 hours post operatively and a middle cerebral artery infarct was diagnosed by CT. Thereafter the patient appeared to have received no further post operative analgesia as all medicines were prescribed orally and the patient was noted by nursing staff to be "too drowsy to swallow".

*Advisors commented that whilst many aspects of this patient's care were exemplary, including clear documentation within the case notes, the lack of administration of even simple analgesics post operatively was unacceptable.*

Anaesthetists completing the questionnaire were not specifically asked whether the need for epidural analgesia influenced choice of ward care. However recent research has demonstrated that this may be the case with a preference for HDU care or extended recovery if an epidural was used.[19] In this study patients having emergency abdominal surgery were less likely to receive epidural analgesia.

In the current sample 28/957 patients received non steroidal anti inflammatory drugs (NSAIDs). Although this is considerably less than in 1999 when 110 patients over 90 years (12%) received NSAIDs, this is still too many. NSAIDs in the elderly are known to have increased gastric and renal complications. Recent reviews have again counselled that they should be used with extreme caution in the elderly.[15] It is concluded that the elderly post operative patient, as with any other age group requires access to effective multimodal analgesia. Training and facilities should be sufficient to support this as a priority within secondary care.

## Organisational issues in delivery of an acute pain service

The organisational questionnaire asked about arrangements for acute pain services (APS).

**Table 6.17 Presence of an Acute Pain Service (APS) in the hospital**

| Acute pain service | n | % |
|---|---|---|
| Yes | 208 | 74.6 |
| No | 71 | 25.4 |
| **Subtotal** | **279** | |
| Not Answered | 4 | |
| **Total** | **283** | |

In 71 hospitals there appeared to be no acute pain service (Table 6.17). The profile of these Trusts is presented in Table 6.18.

**Table 6.18 Absence of acute pain service by hospital type**

| Hospital type | n |
|---|---|
| District General | 6 |
| University Teaching | 4 |
| Community | 6 |
| Limited surgical specialities | 7 |
| Independent | 46 |
| Other | 2 |
| **Total** | **71** |

Most but not all hospitals without an acute pain service were in the independent sector. A further 21 independent hospitals responding to the survey stated that they did have an APS. We also noted that 4 University Hospitals and 6 District General Hospitals (DGHs) apparently had no acute pain service. Single speciality hospitals were relatively highly represented, and we know that some of these were neurosurgical or orthopaedic units.

A 2003 Royal College of Anaesthetists (RCoA) recommendation was for all hospitals to have an APS.[20] A recent detailed report from Australia concluded that there was Grade 3 evidence that the presence of an APS both improves pain relief and reduces incidence of side effects.[15]

Two surveys published in 2004 in the UK [21,22] showed that an APS existed in 83% and 89.4% of hospitals in the UK. However, these surveys did not include the independent sector. It is also possible that questions asked in the organisational questionnaire were ill understood (as definitions of what constitutes an APS vary considerably). In the 1999 study[1] 763/944 (81%) of patients were treated in a hospital with an APS. However in this study as in *Extremes of Age* it was clear that there was a lack of clarity as to what an APS constituted.

If an APS existed, the organisational questionnaire gathered information as to whether the hospital had acute pain nurses (Table 6.19).

**Table 6.19 Designated specialised nurses for the APS**

| Specialist pain nurses | n | % |
|---|---|---|
| Yes | 195 | 93.8 |
| No | 12 | 5.8 |
| Unknown | 1 | <1 |
| **Total** | **208** | |

In 12 Trusts where an acute pain service existed this did not include nursing staff. Whilst different models of an acute pain service have been described, it is difficult to understand how one could function without specialist nursing input. In 1999 it was reported that 629/763 patients were cared for a by a pain team that included specialised pain nurses, and 680/763 by pain teams with consultant input.

Data were therefore collected around funded consultant sessions in acute pain (Table 6.20).

**Table 6.20 Designated funded consultant sessions for the APS**

| Funded consultant sessions | n | % |
|---|---|---|
| Yes | 177 | 86.8 |
| No | 26 | 12.7 |
| Unknown | 1 | <1 |
| **Subtotal** | **204** | |
| Not answered | 4 | |
| **Total** | **208** | |

26 hospitals whilst having an acute pain service did not have funded consultant sessions. There was a spread of different types of institutions, but the independent sector as well as single surgical speciality hospitals were disproportionately represented, and again 9 DGHs and 6 University centres apparently had no funded consultant sessions (Table 6.21).

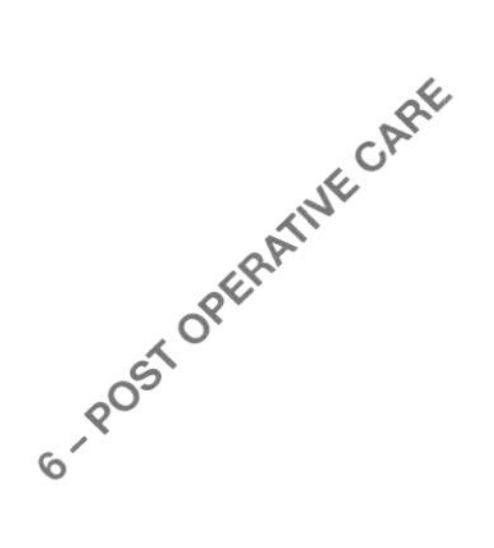


**Table 6.21 Absence of funded consultant sessions by hospital type**

| Hospital type | n |
|---|---|
| District General | 9 |
| University Teaching | 6 |
| Limited surgical specialities | 4 |
| Independent | 6 |
| Other | 1 |
| **Total** | **26** |

If an APS was present data was collected as to what training was provided for staff in the assessment and management of pain in the elderly (Table 6.22).

**Table 6.22 Training provided to ward staff in pain assessment and management in the elderly**

| Training provided in pain assessment | n | % |
|---|---|---|
| Yes | 164 | 83.2 |
| No | 23 | 11.7 |
| Unknown | 10 | 5.1 |
| **Subtotal** | **197** | |
| Not answered | 11 | |
| **Total** | **208** | |

23 hospitals said that they had no specific training in place in the assessment and management of pain in the elderly. Training underpins the effective working of an acute pain service within a Trust. It is disturbing to discover that this was not provided in >10% where elderly patients underwent surgery.

The reasons for lack of implementation of the 1990 UK national recommendations [23] are complex, and have recently been examined.[24] There is no doubt that pre-existing factors at a local level (such as the location of surgical services on many sites, and a lack of ability within organisational infrastructures to adopt a "cross directorate" approach to provision), along with the lack of multidisciplinary consensus on the importance of pain management, have much to do with the lack of implementation of guidance, and contribute to the picture of a patchy and incomplete service which we have identified.

## Key findings

Level 2 and 3 care were generally utilised more than 10 years ago. However it was still planned less often (292/790) than would be expected in view of severity of illness/profile of surgery.

Post operative AKI was related to poor intra-operative management of fluids and cardiovascular status (24/151) and was compounded by deficiencies in post operative management.

Particular skills and knowledge are required in assessing and treating pain in the elderly. Pain was not assessed routinely post operatively in all the elderly surgical patients included in this study (135/612).

Continuous infusion based analgesia (such as epidurals and patient controlled analgesia) was used relatively sparingly in this population.

A substantial number of hospitals still do not have acute pain teams (71/279), and many of these are in the independent sector. Those that do may not have funded consultant sessions, nurses or programmes of training.

## Recommendations

There is an ongoing need for provision of peri-operative level 2 and 3 care to support major surgery in the elderly, particularly for those with comorbidity. For less major surgery extended recovery and high observation facilities in existing wards should be considered. (Commissioning Leads, Trusts, Clinical Directors)

Post operative Acute Kidney Injury (AKI) is avoidable in the elderly and should not occur. There is a need for continuous postgraduate education of physicians, surgeons and anaesthetists around the assessment of risk factors for the development of AKI in the elderly surgical patient. (Postgraduate Deans, Medical Directors)

Fluid management must be clearly documented, and form part of the routine review and handover between theatres and wards. This should continue on at least a daily basis thereafter, alongside monitoring of biochemical function. (Consultants, Nurses)

Pain is the 5th vital sign, and requires the same status as heart rate and blood pressure in the assessment and management of all patients. Clear and specific guidance on the recognition and treatment of pain in the elderly should be incorporated into education programmes. (Clinical Directors, Postgraduate Deans, Trusts)

A fully resourced acute pain service (APS) is essential within the context of modern secondary care services. This includes the Independent Sector. (Clinical Directors)

***References***


1. National Confidential Enquiry into Patient Outcome and Death. *Extremes of Age, The 1999 report of the National Confidential Enquiry into Peri-operative Death*. 1999. NCEPOD, London

2. Department of Health. Critical care beds. http://www.dh.gov.uk/en/Publicationsandstatistics/Statistics/Performancedataandstatistics/Beds/DH_077451. Last modified 26th August 2010. Crown Copyright

3. Department of Health. *Quality Critical Care: Beyond 'Comprehensive Critical Care': A report by the Critical Care Stakeholder Forum*. Crown Copyright

4. ICNARC case mix programme-case mix and outcome summary statistics, April 2008 - March 2009. www.icnarc.org

5. Pisani MA. Analytic Reviews: Considerations in caring for the critically ill older patients. *Journal of Intensive Care Medicine.* 2009; 24(2), 83 - 95

6. Department of Health. *National Service Framework for older people*. 2001. Crown Copyright

7. Preston SD, Ashley RD et al. Geriatric surgery is about diseases not age. *Journal of the Royal Society of Medicine.* 2008; 101, 409 - 415

8. Ford PNR, Thomas I et al. Determinants of outcome in critically ill octogenarians after surgery: An observational study. *British Journal of Anaesthesia.* 2007; 99(6), 824 - 829

9. Farfel JM, Franca SA et al. Age, invasive ventilatory support and outcomes in elderly patients admitted to intensive care units. *Age and Ageing.* 2009; 38(5), 515 - 20

10. Hennessy D, Juzwishin K et al. Outcomes of elderly survivors of intensive care. *Chest.* 2005; 127(5), 1764 - 1774

11. McGory ML, Kao KK et al. Developing Quality indicators for elderly surgical patients. *Annals of Surgery*. 2009; 250(2), 338 - 347.

12. National Confidential Enquiry into Patient Outcome and Death. *Caring to the End?* 2009. NCEPOD, London

13. National Confidential Enquiry into Patient Outcome and Death. *Acute kidney Injury: Adding insult to injury.* 2009. NCEPOD, London

14. Healthcare Commission. *Caring for Dignity. A national report on dignity in care for older people while in hospital.* 2007. Commission for Healthcare and Audit

15. Australian and New Zealand College of Anaesthetist and Faculty of Pain Medicine. *Acute Pain Management - Scientific Evidence.* 2010. 3rd Edition, NHMRC. Australian and New Zealand College of Anaesthetists

16. Morrison SR, Magaziner J et al. Relationship between pain and opioid analgesics on the development of delirium following hip fracture. *Journals of Gerontology Series A.* 2003; 58(1), M76 - M881

17. Royal College of Anaesthetists, Royal College of Nursing, Association of Anaesthetists, British Pain Society and the European Society of Regional Anaesthesia and Pain Therapy. *Good practice in the management of continuous epidural analgesia in the hospital setting.* 2004. Royal College of Anaesthetists, Royal College of Nursing, Association of Anaesthetists, British Pain Society and the European Society of Regional Anaesthesia and Pain Therapy

18. Gagliese L, Jackson M et al. Age is not an impediment to the use of patient-controlled analgesia by surgical patients. *Anesthesiology.* 2000; 93(3), 601 - 610

19. Walton B, Farrow C & Cook TM. A national survey of epidural use and management in elderly patients undergoing elective and emergency laparotomy. *Anaesthesia.* 2006; 61(10), 456 - 461

20. Royal College of Anaesthetists. P*ain Management Services, Good Practice.* 2003. Royal College of Anaesthetists

21. Powell AE, Davies HTO et al. Rhetoric and reality on acute pain services in the UK: a national postal questionnaire survey. *British Journal of Anaesthesia.* 2004; 92(5), 689 - 693

22. Nagi H. Acute Pain Services in the United Kingdom. *Acute Pain.* 2004; 5, 89 - 107

23. The Royal College of Surgeons of England. *Report of the Working Party on Pain after Surgery.* 1990. Royal College of Surgeons of England

24. Powell AE, Davies HT et al. Understanding the challenges of service change - learning from acute pain services in the UK. *Journal of the Royal Society of Medicine.* 2009; 102(2), 62-68

# 7 – Summary

## General findings

During the process of peer review of the records, Advisors were encouraged to provide written details where they identified specific remediable factors in the process of care. They did so in a total of 302 cases. The most commonly recurring themes are tabulated below (Table 7.1). There was often overlap between these broad categories, for example the wrong level of seniority frequently led to delay, due to poor pre-operative preparation and poor decision making. Poor team structures and lack of Medicine for the Care of Older People (MCOP) input was often associated with lack of optimisation and delay.

In 17 cases it was thought that aggressive surgery had been undertaken, but no provision for appropriate levels of after-care had been made. Post operative care in general was often managed by junior members of the team, and there was often poor communication and failure to involve more senior staff or other specialties when it would have been appropriate to do so.

Poor fluid management and poor documentation continue to be highlighted by Advisors. There were a small number of cases when analgesic regimens were believed to be poor.

**Table 7.1 Recurring themes of concern identified by Advisors within the whole study sample**

| Recurring themes | n* |
|---|---|
| Seniority | 67 |
| Team structure | 70 |
| MCOP input | 29 |
| Decision making | 84 |
| Delay | 54 |
| Pre-operative preparation | 105 |
| Failure to optimise patient | 30 |
| Post operative care | 53 |
| Aggressive surgery without after care | 17 |
| Poor fluid resuscitation | 21 |
| Poor communication | 39 |
| Consent | 15 |
| Poor documentation | 71 |
| Poor analgesia | 7 |

**answers may be multiple*

Chapters 7.1 and 7.2 will concentrate upon the care of patients admitted within the two most common diagnostic groups, fractured neck of femur and the acute abdomen. Within these two sub chapters we will explore the general findings already discussed in the main body of the report but specialty groups may be particularly interested in the analysis of these cases.

# 7.1 – Care of fractured neck of femur

As previously stated the UK has a rapidly expanding population of elderly people; in line with this hip fracture in the older person is becoming more frequent. In 2007 70,000 people suffered a hip fracture and that number is increasing 2% per annum. This represents a major burden on the health care system and in financial terms is estimated to cost the National Health Service (NHS) about £1.8 billion. The 30 day peri-operative mortality rate is 10% and this rises to 30% within 1 year. Concurrent comorbidities and multiple medications complicate management contributing to delays in surgery, post operative mobilisation and hospital discharge. Given that in this study, over a third of patients underwent surgery for a fractured neck of femur (fractured NOF), it is appropriate that the care of this group of patients be examined in greater detail.

## Existing standards and guidelines

The British Orthopaedic Association (BOA) has produced a standards document for the management of hip fracture in the older person.[1]

These standards specify *inter alia*:

- Admission to an appropriate ward area within 4 hours
- Recognition of analgesic needs bearing in mind the high level of cognitive impairment
- Avoiding pre-operative dehydration
- Assessing risk and avoiding pressure area problems
- Surgical fixation should not be delayed for more than 48 hours unless there are clear reversible medical conditions
- There should be an appropriate composition and seniority of the surgical team
- Antibiotic prophylaxis should be administered.
- Orthogeriatricians should be involved in ***all stages*** of care.[1]

Guidance in the National Service Framework (NSF) for Older People suggests that surgery for fractured NOF should be performed with 24 hours of admission.[2]

It is clear from this study that not all of these standards are being met.

In this study (where a surgical questionnaire was returned) 383/1120 (34.2%) were admitted with a diagnosis of fracture NOF, and 424/1120 (37.9%) of patients underwent surgery for a fractured NOF. The difference is accounted for by patients admitted with either an incorrect initial diagnosis, multiple diagnoses, or patients who fell sustaining a fracture whilst an in-patient for another condition. Case notes were only returned for 306 patients who underwent surgery for fractured NOF.

## Initial assessment following admission

The majority of patients who underwent a procedure for a fractured neck of femur were first assessed on arrival and following their admission by basic grades of doctor (Figure 7.1.1, Figure 7.1.2).

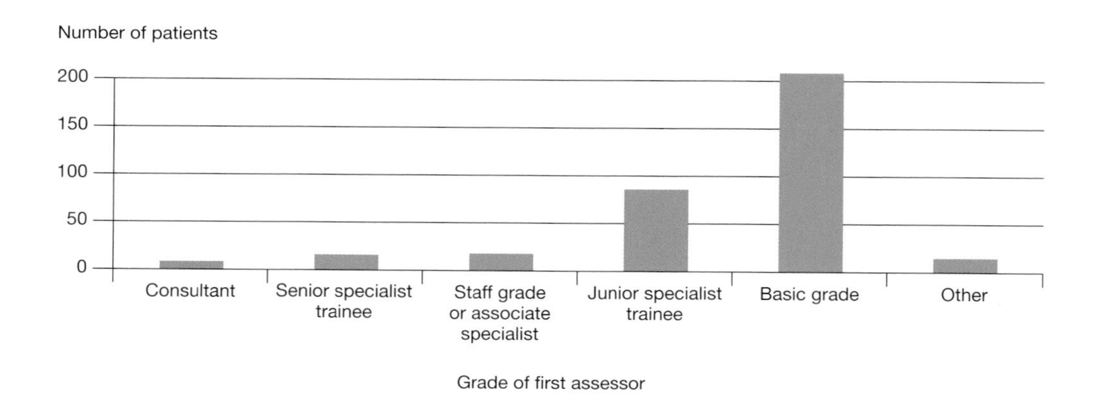


**Figure 7.1.1. Grade of first assessor on arrival**

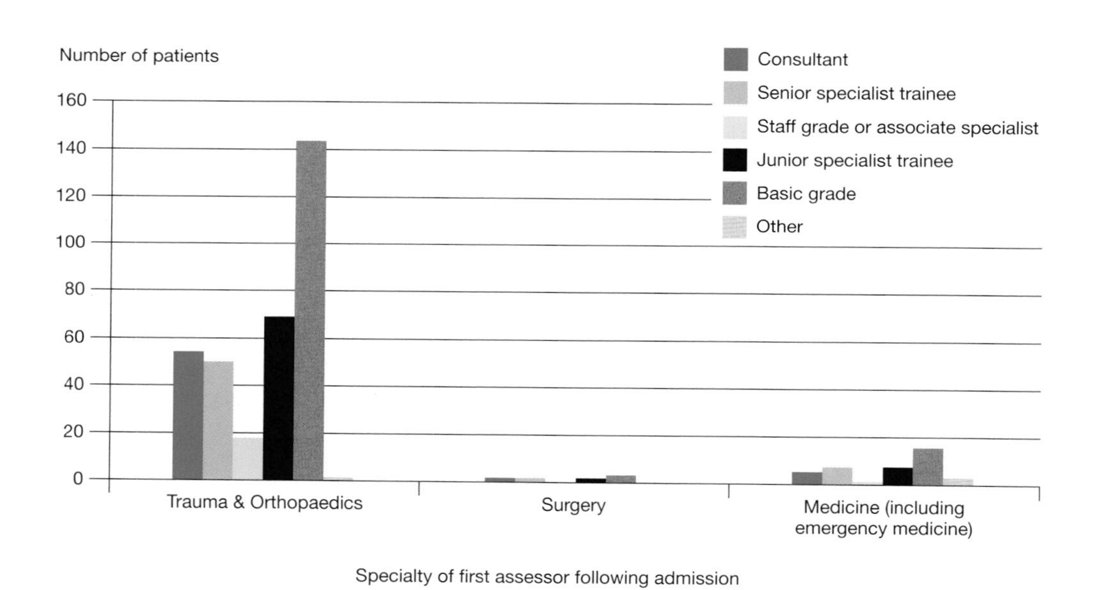


**Figure 7.1.2. Grade and specialty of first assessor following admission**

## Appropriateness of first assessment

**Table 7.1.1 Appropriateness of the time, grade and specialty of the initial assessment compared to the severity and complexity of the illness – Advisors' opinion**

| Appropriateness of first assessment | n | % |
|---|---|---|
| Yes | 278 | 97.9 |
| No | 6 | 2.1 |
| **Subtotal** | **284** | |
| Unable to answer | 20 | |
| Not answered | 2 | |
| **Total** | **306** | |

Despite the preponderance of initial assessment being performed by basic grades, Advisors were mainly of the view that this was appropriate (Table 7.1.1). There was some dissent from the MCOP Advisors, who believed that earlier senior MCOP assessment might assist in timely optimisation and minimise the delay to operation.

The Royal College of Surgeons of England[3] has recently published a policy statement, which advocates consultant delivered rather than consultant led care. These data indicate that this is not currently happening for patients admitted with a fractured neck of femur. Orthopaedic Advisors were of the opinion that it is appropriate for this initial specialty assessment to be undertaken by basic grade staff, as the assessment and diagnosis of a fractured femur is usually straight forward. However most of these elderly patients had significant comorbidities, and the recognition of these, subsequent optimisation, treatment planning and decision making requires senior input.

Consultant review could only be identified by the Advisors from the clinical records in just over half of the cases (Table 7.1.2).

**Table 7.1.2 Time, date and location of the first consultant review identified from the notes – Advisors' opinion**

| Consultant review identified | n | % |
|---|---|---|
| Yes | 145 | 51.1 |
| No | 139 | 48.9 |
| **Subtotal** | **284** | |
| Unable to answer | 21 | |
| Not answered | 1 | |
| **Total** | **306** | |

**Table 7.1.3 Evidence of a delay in consultant review – Advisors' opinion**

| Delay in consultant review | n | % |
|---|---|---|
| Yes | 32 | 15.2 |
| No | 178 | 84.8 |
| **Subtotal** | **210** | |
| Unable to answer | 90 | |
| Not answered | 6 | |
| **Total** | **306** | |

Bearing in mind the difficulty that Advisors encountered in identifying the point at which consultants were involved, they were nonetheless able to positively identify a delay in consultant review which was of clinical significance in 15% of cases (Table 7.1.3).

The surgeons indicated that even in trauma and orthopaedics, where there are some funded sessions for orthogeriatricians, the direct input into patient care by specialist consultant physicians occurred in only 41.9% of cases (Table 7.1.4). Eight cases who went on to have an operation for fractured NOF were admitted under MCOP.

**Table 7.1.4 Review by an MCOP consultant If not admitted under MCOP**

| Review by MCOP | n | % |
|---|---|---|
| Yes | 161 | 41.9 |
| No | 183 | 47.7 |
| Unknown | 40 | 10.4 |
| **Subtotal** | **384** | |
| Not answered | 32 | |
| **Total** | **416** | |

The following case study presents an example of lack of MCOP involvement.

**Case study 20**

A patient admitted with a fractured NOF was admitted also suffered from dementia, IHD and previous CVAs. Their Glasgow Coma Score reduced during admission from 15 to 13. This was not investigated, and there was no input from MCOP. In the post operative period it was noted that on admission they had been in atrial fibrillation and death occurred on day 3 post operation of a presumed embolic stroke.

*Advisors thought that had a physician been involved from the outset, management of the comorbdities might have prevented this complication.*

In the majority of cases where there was regular input from MCOP to the surgical team, this input was limited to a weekly ward round, and indeed it was notable that few MCOP teams were involved in the production of policies and procedures for the management of elderly patients (Table 7.1.5).

**Table 7.1.5 Constitution of formal input from MCOP to the surgical team**

| MCOP input to the surgical team | n* |
|---|---|
| Weekly ward round | 212 |
| Input into guidelines and policies | 88 |
| On call service only/referral service | 95 |
| Other | 128 |

**answers may be multiple*

Given that there is a clear recognition of the survival advantage of early optimisation followed by timely operation for this group of patients, a weekly ward round would not appear to provide the level of involvement appropriate for most patients, as envisaged by the NSF.

The ultimate decision to operate was usually undertaken by a consultant (353/414, 85.3%), but there was not usually evidence that the consultant had reviewed the patient in the notes, before surgery. The grade of clinician making the decision to operate was not answered in 10 cases.

The decision to operate was therefore largely being undertaken by consultants based on the clinical assessment and information gathered by junior staff. Orthopaedic Advisors were of the view that this was largely appropriate, because the diagnosis of a fractured femur is straight forward on clinical and radiological grounds. It was suggested that far more orthopaedic trauma operations are now undertaken by consultants, and this is because job plans increasingly make provision for them to undertake planned trauma theatre lists. Nonetheless, the diagnosis of complex medical comorbidities, and the assessment of their relevance in the overall context of care of these sick elderly patients, was sometimes not best served by this model of care.

In the 1999 Extremes of Age report[4] NCEPOD noted that orthopaedic surgeons need to establish whether there was sufficient expertise available within the team to manage the complex medical problems of elderly patients, and pointed out the seniority of surgeons and anaesthetists should be determined by the physical status of the patient and not just the orthopaedic diagnosis or procedure required.

## Delays

The first assessment after arrival at hospital was usually timely as shown in the Figure below where over 90% of patients were assessed within 4 hours of admission. (Figure 7.1.3)

However surgeons completing the questionnaire reported a delay between admission and surgery in over 44% of cases (Table 7.1.6).

**Table 7.1.6 Delays between admission and surgery**

| Delays between admission and surgery | n | % |
|---|---|---|
| Yes | 185 | 44.4 |
| No | 227 | 54.4 |
| Unknown | 5 | 1.2 |
| **Subtotal** | **417** | |
| Not answered | 7 | |
| **Total** | **424** | |

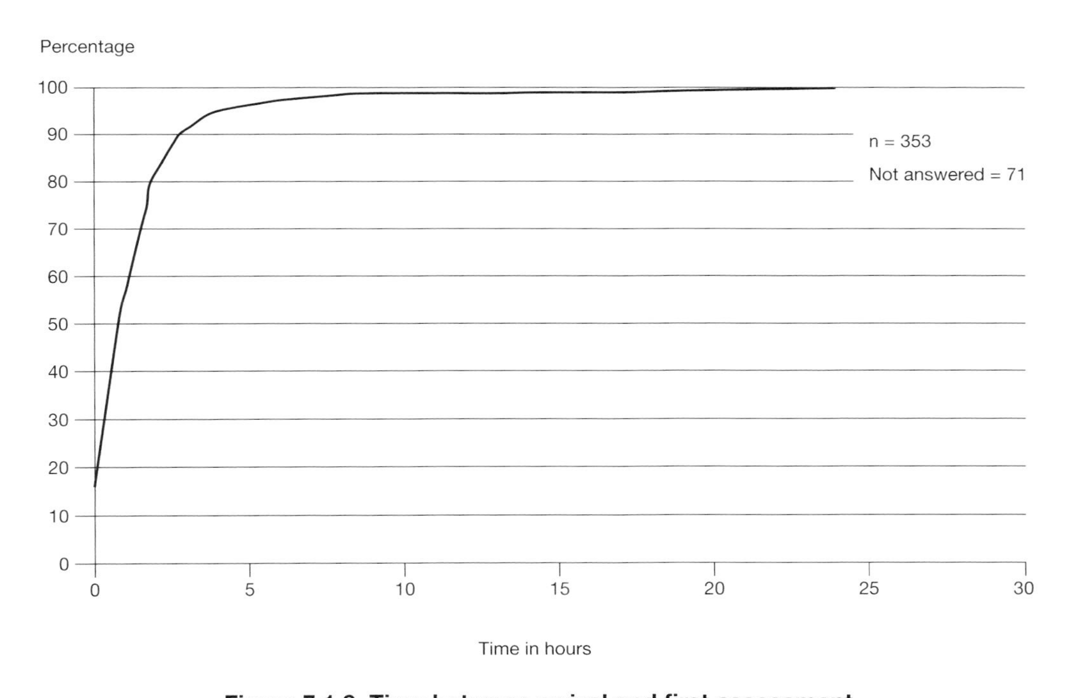


**Figure 7.1.3. Time between arrival and first assessment**

BOA[1] and NSF[2] guidance recommends that patients should undergo surgery within 48 hours or 24 hours (once medically fit) respectively. As stated above, there was a delay between admission and operation in 185/417 patients who underwent an operation for fractured neck of femur. The surgeon completing the questionnaire was asked how many days surgery was delayed by. Where there was a delay between admission and operation, in 53/143 (37%) of patients there was a delay of 1 day, and in 25 (13%) patients there was a delay of 5 days or more days (Figure 7.1.4). In 42 patients the length of delay was not quantified. Unfortunately, no further information was gathered as to the cause of the delay.

This is a complex issue. The judgement about when a patient is optimised for surgery and when the risks and benefits of further delay against potential further optimisation requires considerable expertise. It is very difficult to establish whether patients who wait > 48 hours for surgery do so because of inferior systems of care or because comorbidity precludes early surgery.[5,6]

The view of the surgeons and anaesthetists involved in the cases is not always the same. As previously noted from the anaesthetic questionnaire, a high proportion of delays are ascribed by anaesthetists to a delay in the decision to operate, rather than necessary delays in order to optimise the patient (Table 4.6 Chapter 4).

Perhaps the best assessment of clinically significant delay in this group comes from the global assessment of the Advisors. In their opinion the operation was not conducted in a timely way in just over 28% of cases (Table 7.1.7). This was often because of lack of appropriate clinical expertise and communication with senior staff in the early phase of admission.

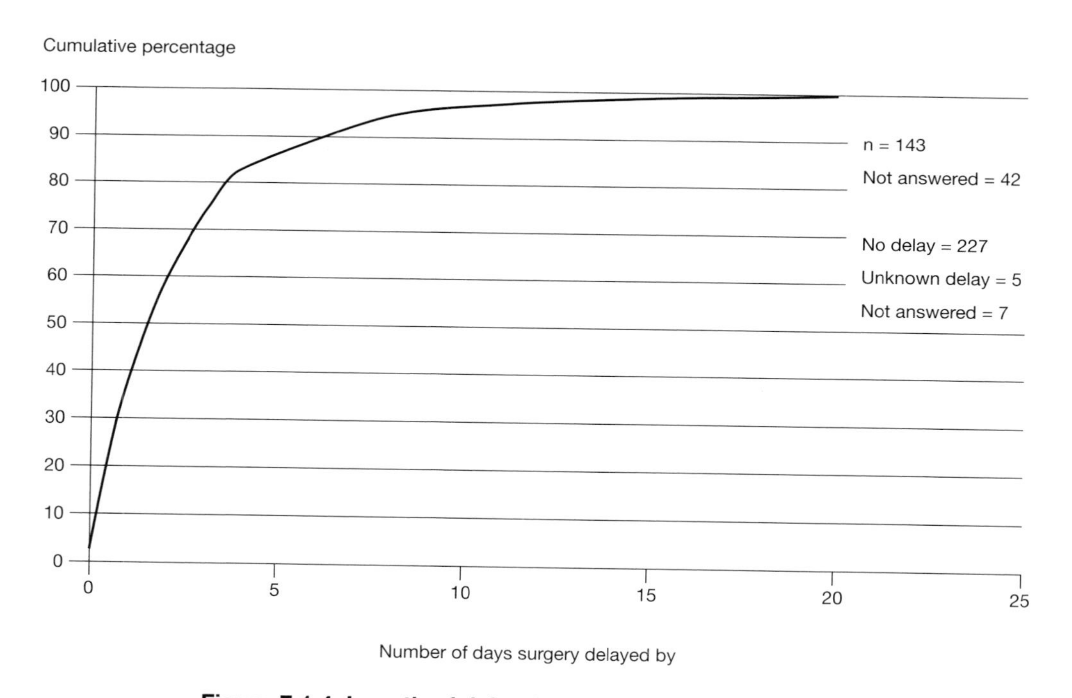


**Figure 7.1.4. Length of delay from admission to operation**

**Table 7.1.7 Timeliness of the operation performed – Advisors' opinion**

| Operation performed in a timely manner | n | % |
|---|---|---|
| Yes | 215 | 71.2 |
| No | 87 | 28.8 |
| **Subtotal** | **302** | |
| Unable to answer | 4 | |
| **Total** | **306** | |

Case study 21 demonstrates an example of delays in operating.

**Case study 21**

A patient admitted with fractured NOF developed a chest infection within 48 hrs of admission. Operation was delayed whilst attempts were made to optimise the patient's respiratory function without input from any MCOP or other physicians. Following surgery the patient died of pneumonia.

*As per Scottish Intercollegiate Guidelines Network (SIGN) guidelines[7], chasing unrealistic medical goals such as pulmonary infections, which delays surgery, is not usually appropriate. A more experienced physician would be more likely to be familiar with this evidence.*

**Case study 22**

A wheelchair bound patient was transferred from another hospital for deteriorating bronchiectasis. During the transfer the patient had fallen. On admission the patient was noted to have pressure sores and was MRSA positive. The patient's pain and immobility was attributed to pre-existing arthritis and pressure sores. Two weeks after admission a radiograph demonstrated a fractured NOF. The patient died of pneumonia 10 days after surgery.

*Advisors were of the view, that any elderly patient falling, and with hip pain, particularly if there were signs of external rotation, should be suspected of having a fracture, and referred for an orthopaedic opinion.*

### Failure to seek advice by juniors

**Table 7.1.8 Evidence that junior staff did not seek appropriate advice when necessary – Advisors' opinion**

| Seeking appropriate advice | n | % |
|---|---|---|
| Yes | 66 | 23.6 |
| No | 214 | 76.4 |
| **Subtotal** | **280** | |
| Unable to answer | 25 | |
| Not answered | 1 | |
| **Total** | **306** | |

The previously cited examples of inexperienced doctors failing to seek advice are by no means isolated, indeed in almost a quarter of patients undergoing an operation for a fractured NOF Advisors judged that junior clinicians did not seek appropriate advice from consultants when they should have done (Table 7.1.8). The reasons for this are unclear, however one of the problems could be that inexperience leads to a recognition of when help is required.

### ASA Grade

Whilst there were fewer patients in the ASA grades 4-5 than in the general surgery group, the majority of patients with fractured neck of femur were still ASA 3 or greater on admission (Figure 7.1.5). This re-enforces the point that most of the elderly patients studied who died following fractured NOF had a high level of physical impairment, and therefore should have received the benefit of input from appropriately experienced clinicians.

### Venous Thromboembolism Risk Assessment

**Table 7.1.9 Appropriate risk assessment for thrombotic complications – Advisors' opinion**

| Appropriate risk assessment for thrombosis | n | % |
|---|---|---|
| Yes | 201 | 80.4 |
| No | 49 | 19.6 |
| **Subtotal** | **250** | |
| Unable to answer | 51 | |
| Not answered | 5 | |
| **Total** | **306** | |

20% of patients where Advisors were able to make an assessment were judged not to have been appropriately risk assessed for venous thromboembolism (VTE) (Table 7.1.9). Whilst this is better than in previous

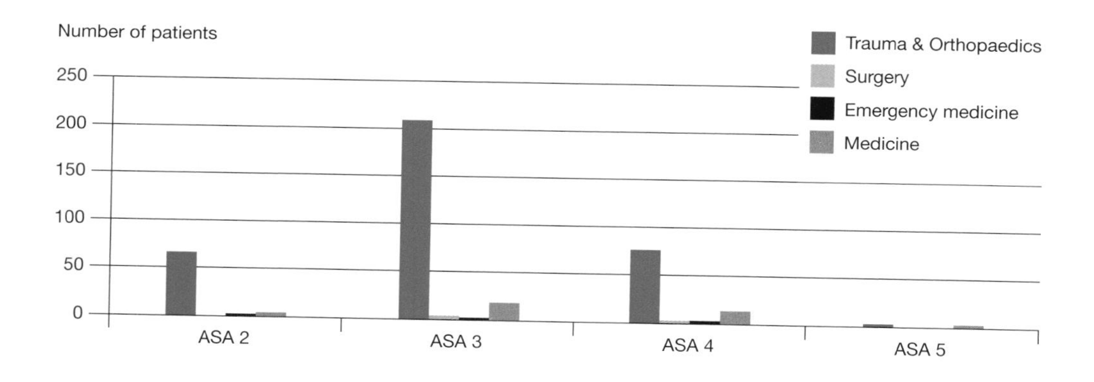


**Figure 7.1.5. Health status on admission by the specialty of the clinician the patient was first admitted to**

NCEPOD studies, it still would not achieve The Quality, Innovation, Productivity and Prevention (QIPP) target[8], and this would translate into financial penalties, for those institutions failing to undertake and record an appropriate risk assessment in 90% of cases. Whilst it should be noted that QIPP had not been conceived and the National Institute for Clinical Health and Excellence (NICE) guidelines for orthopaedics[9] had not been ratified at the time of this study, the value of VTE risk assessment and prophylaxis was well recognised and the subject of a previous NCEPOD reports.[10]

### Skin viability

**Table 7.1.10 Assessment of skin viability**

| Skin viability assessed | n | % |
|---|---|---|
| Yes | 238 | 59.9 |
| No | 27 | 6.8 |
| Unknown | 132 | 33.2 |
| **Subtotal** | **397** | |
| Not answered | 27 | |
| **Total** | **424** | |

Evidence of skin viability assessment having been undertaken could not be found in about 33% of cases, and in 7% of cases assessment was not done (Table 7.1.10). This was noted with concern, given the very high risk for elderly patients who are immobile following fractured neck of femur, and the particular risks of infection that pressure sores pose, where hip prostheses have been inserted.

### Antibiotic prophylaxis

The majority of patients undergoing surgery for fractured neck of femur received prophylactic antibiotics; a small number did not (Table 7.1.11). Advisors did not consider that there was any justification for omitting prophylactic antibiotics in patients undergoing surgery for repair of fractured neck of femur.

**Table 7.1.11 Administration of antibiotics to cover the operation**

| Antibiotics administered | n | % |
|---|---|---|
| Yes | 394 | 96.1 |
| No | 6 | 1.5 |
| Unknown | 10 | 2.4 |
| **Subtotal** | **410** | |
| Not answered | 14 | |
| **Total** | **424** | |

### Seniority

The grade of the most senior operating surgeon is shown in Figure 7.1.6. As can be seen only about one third of the fractured neck of femur cases were performed by consultants, and about one third by senior specialist trainees and a third by staff grade and associate specialist (SAS) grades. The number of operations being performed by SAS grades has not noticeably changed since the 1999 report. Whilst far fewer procedures are being undertaken by basic grade Senior House Officers (SHOs) now, if one groups the junior specialist trainees in with the basic grades (the level of a senior SHO in 1999 probably equates to a junior specialist trainee in this study period), then the proportion of cases being undertaken by junior grades has probably not changed in the last 11 years.

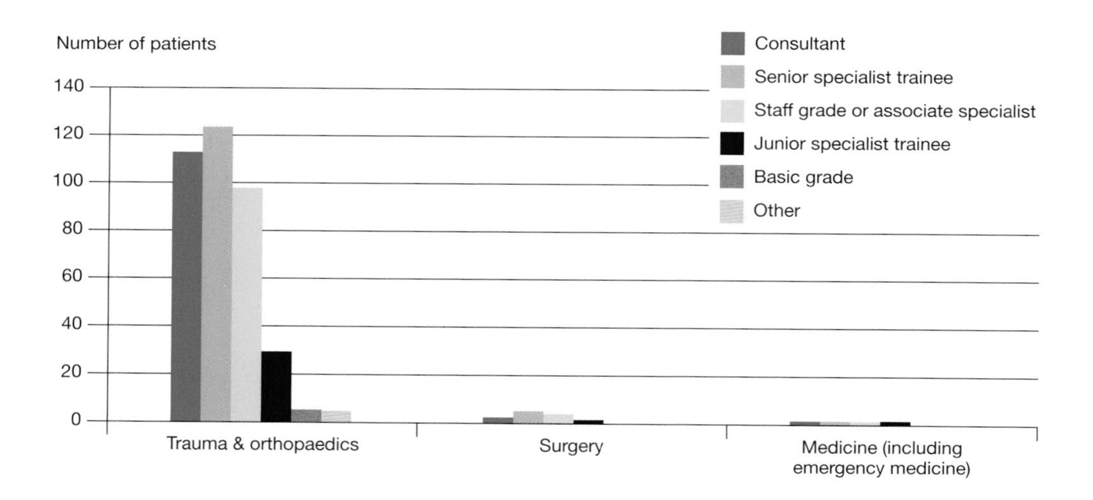


**Figure 7.1.6. Specialty of the most senior operating surgeon by the grade of the most senior clinician proposing the operation**

Where both the surgical questionnaire and case notes were returned (n=263), Advisors were asked to assess whether a trainee was present in theatre when a consultant was operating. A consultant performed the operation in 71 cases. In 48/55 where a consultant was operating a trainee was present in theatre. In 7 cases the Advisor was unable to answer the question, in 4 cases they did not answer the question, and in 5 cases they indicated the question was not applicable. A more junior doctor was operating in 185 cases and it was unknown which grade of surgeon carried out the procedure in 7 cases.

Where the consultant was not operating, the Advisors were asked to assess whether supervision was appropriate. In the majority of cases where Advisors were able to make an assessment, (82/93) they judged that the level of supervision for trainees was appropriate to their grade, but in 11/93 there was judged to have been inadequate supervision. Advisors were unable to answer the question in 71 cases and did not answer the question in 21. In 23.6% (66/280) of cases Advisors judged that trainee surgeons and/or anaesthetists had failed to seek consultant advice when appropriate in a proportion of cases.

## The anaesthetic

Within the group of patients undergoing an operation for a fracture NOF, 40 patients underwent general anaesthetic alone, 152 regional or neuraxial block with GA or sedation and 68 underwent unsupplemented spinal anaesthesia, with or without a nerve block. All ASA grades received all types of anaesthesia with no clear preference demonstrated (Figure 7.1.7).

The most frequently used anaesthetic was therefore a nerve or regional block with either general anaesthesia or sedation.

A recent review of more than 2000 cases of surgery for NOF from 22 centres, looked specifically at the type of anaesthetic administered, and reported that about half the patients received general anaesthetic, and the other half a regional technique.[11] This lack of preference reflects the fact that there is no clear evidence that mortality is affected by type of anaesthetic in this population. A Cochrane review published in 2004[12] concluded that there was "insufficient evidence to rule out clinically important differences".

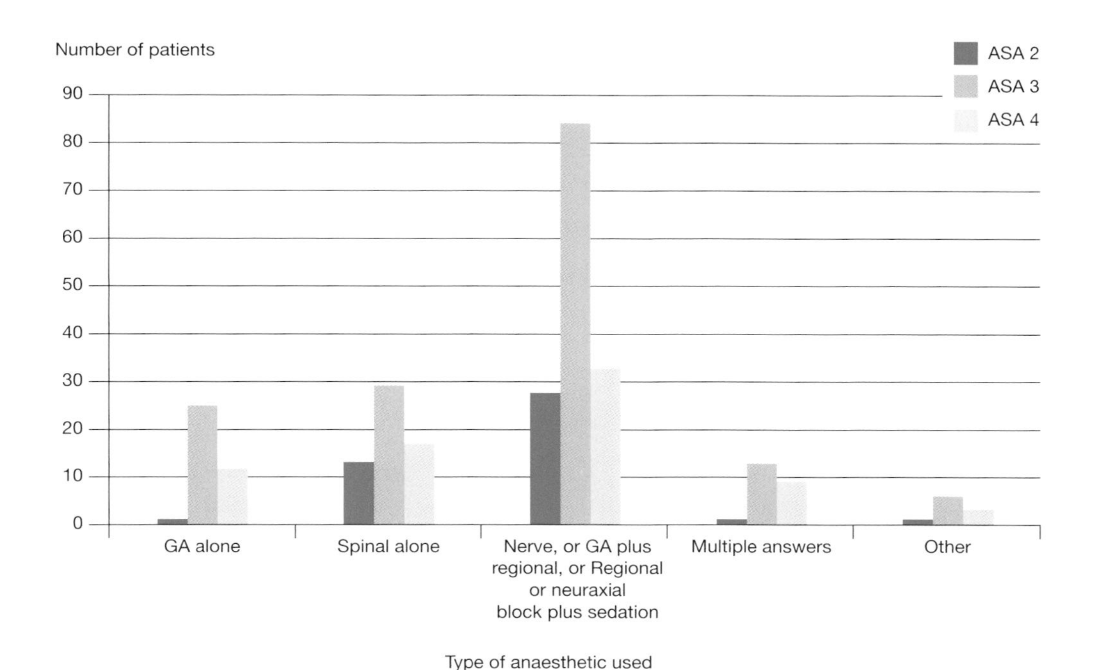


**Figure 7.1.7. Type of anaesthetic used by ASA grade prior to surgery**

However there is evidence of a possible benefit to regional versus general anaesthesia in the elderly with dementia with regard to post operative confusion and cognitive deficit[13], which may have long term deleterious effects.[14] There is also increasing evidence to suggest that general anaesthesia may worsen outcome in patients with dementia.[15,16]

The UK hip fracture anaesthesia network[17] hopes to provide definitive evidence to guide anaesthetic practice in the future.

## Post operative care

Advisors observed that the post operative management of patients was being frequently undertaken by basic grade doctors in orthopaedics, without evidence of senior input or input from MCOP; the following case study presents such an example.

**Case study 23**

A patient had an uncomplicated operation to repair a fractured NOF. However during the post operative period there was no evidence of medical review for 5 days, during which time the observation charts indicated that the patient was becoming increasingly unwell. The nursing notes recorded that the patient was not eating and was complaining of abdominal pain. Eventually a basic grade orthopaedic doctor saw the patient and simply noted an increased respiratory rate and hypotension. There was no senior input, and eventually the patient died of an ischaemic bowel.

*Advisors were of the view that the junior trainees had failed to recognise the seriousness of this patient's illness.*

## Key findings

In 87/302 of cases there was considered to be a clinically significant delay between admission and operation. Delays were still frequent between admission and operation for patients included in this study with fractured NOF, despite BOA and NSF guidelines. Advisors reported a delay in 87/302 cases.

In the opinion of the Advisors trainees did not always seek advice from consultants when this was indicated (66/280 cases).

Initial assessment, and treatment planning was often left to basic grade clinicians.

Pre-operative optimisation of patients did not always occur in a timely manner in the patients included in this study.

The orthopaedic trauma service still relies heavily on trainees and SAS doctors.

Direct input into individual patient care by consultants in MCOP was relatively rare.

Post operative care was often delegated to junior orthopaedic trainees.

## Recommendations

The British Orthopaedic Association and The British Geriatric Society should provide more specific guidance on the ideal levels of seniority and speciality input into the assessment and decision making phase of the care pathway for patients with fractured neck of femur. (British Orthopaedic Association, British Geriatrics Society)

The decision about when a patient's physical condition is optimised and when to operate in patients with fractured neck of femur is critical, and requires multi-disciplinary input and expertise. There must be senior surgical, medical and anaesthetic input at this point in the care pathway. (Clinical Directors, Consultants)

***References***


1. British Orthopaedic Association Standards for Trauma (BOAST) 1. *Hip Fracture in the Older Person.* 2008. British Orthopaedic Association

2. Department of Health. *National Service Framework for older people.* 2001. Crown Copyright

3. Royal College of Surgeons of England. *The consultant surgeon and consultant delivered service position statement.* 2010. RCS England

4. National Confidential Enquiry into Patient Outcome and Death. *Extremes of Age, The 1999 report of the National Confidential Enquiry into Peri-operative Death.* 1999. NCEPOD, London

5. Bryson G. Waiting for hip fracture repair – Do outcomes and patients suffer? *Canadian Journal of Anaesthesiology.* 2008; 55(3), 135 - 139

6. Shiga T et al. Is operative delay associated with increased mortality of hip fracture patients? Systematic review, meta-analysis and meta-regression. *Canadian Journal of Anaesthesiology.* 2008; 55(3), 146 - 154

7. Scottish Intercollegiate Guidelines Network. *Management of hip fracture in older people. A national clinical guideline.* 2009. Scottish Intercollegiate Guidelines Network

8. Best Practice Tariff (BPT) for Fragility Hip Fracture Care. Department of Health 2010. http://webarchive.nationalarchives.gov.uk/+/www.dh.gov.uk/en/Managingyourorganisation/Financeandplanning/NHSFinancialReforms/DH_105080

9. National Institute for Health and Clinical Excellence. Venous thromboembolism; reducing the risk of venous thromboembolism in inpatients undergoing surgery. 2007.

10. National Confidential Enquiry into Patient Outcome and Death. *Caring to the end?* 2009. NCEPOD, London

11. White SM, Griffiths R et al. Anaesthesia for proximal femoral fracture in the UK: first report from the NHS Hip Fracture Anaesthesia network. *Anaesthesia.* 2010; 65(3), 243 - 248

12. Parker MJ, Handoll HHG & Griffiths R. Anaesthesia for hip fracture surgery in adults. Cochrane database of Systematic Reviews. 2004; 4. John Wiley & Sons, Ltd.

13. Fodale V, Quattrone D et al. Alzheimer's disease and anaesthesia: implications for the central cholinergic system. *British Journal of Anaesthesia.* 2006; 97, 445 - 52

14. Steinmetz J, Christensen KB et al. Long-term consequences of post operative cognitive dysfunction. *Anaesthesiology.* 2009. 110(3), 548 - 555

15. Harris AR & Eger E. Alzheimer's disease and anaesthesia: Out of body, out of mind...or not? *Annals of Neurology*. 2008; 64(6), 597 - 599

16. Tang J, Eckenhoff MF & Eckenhoff RG. Anaesthesia and the old brain. *Anaesthesia and Analgesia*. 2010; 110(2), 421 - 426

17. National Health Service. Hip *Fracture Anaesthesia*. 2010. http://www.networks.nhs.uk/nhs-networks/hip-fracture-anaesthesia. NHS Networks. Last accessed 15th September 2010

# 7.2 – Care of the acute abdomen

Patients aged 80 and above have a high incidence of chronic medical illness, particularly cardio-respiratory and cerebro-vascular disease, diabetes, renal impairment and poor mobility. Despite our awareness of these issues there is little data describing outcomes for octogenarians undergoing emergency laparotomy. That such patients have a high morbidity and mortality was first confirmed in a Danish population study published by Madsen (1993) which showed a 39% mortality for this cohort.[1] Two more recent studies have reported mortality rates of 42% for emergency general surgery[2] and 32% for emergency colorectal surgery.[3] Another study has also shown mortality rates of 10-55% for older patients (>65 yr) undergoing urgent or emergency colorectal surgery.[4]

An earlier study provides compelling evidence of the impact of delays in proceeding to laparotomy in these elderly patients with death rates increasing from 6% to 45% when surgery took place more than 24 hours after admission.[5]

There is often debate about the appropriateness of surgery in elderly patients with an acute abdominal catastrophe and major comorbidities.[4] Nevertheless a small study by Church (2005) showed that 14/21 moribund patients (ASA 5) from a cohort of 2040 survived 30 days and 7/21 (2/4 aged >80) were discharged from hospital.[6] This emphasises the difficulty of denying surgery to these sick patients particularly given the lack of a robust risk assessment method for predicting outcomes.

Whilst it might be expected that modern standards of care should improve outcomes this may not always be the case. In particular invasive medical management may undermine the broader care of patients. This was highlighted recently by Toulson, Davisson & Correia (2009) who found that the risk of malnutrition in patients undergoing major abdominal surgery remains prevalent despite other advances in care.[7]

This chapter examines a number of aspects of the care of patients undergoing emergency surgery on the acute abdomen.

## Outcomes

285 patients were admitted with an "acute abdomen" and subsequently died, 239 of whom underwent intra-peritoneal abdominal surgery. This includes patients who underwent either abdominal surgery or bowel resection for a strangulated hernia. In the other 50 cases death occurred following a variety of procedures, the most common of which were upper gastrointestinal endoscopy/endoscopic retrograde cholangiopancreatography for gastrointestinal haemorrhage or hepatobiliary disease (n = 24) and insertion of a colonic stent (n = 5).

A further 35 patients died following surgery on their abdomen who were not considered to have acute abdominal pathology at the time of admission, but who subsequently underwent surgery for an acute abdomen. Whilst some of these patients developed an inter-current illness (originally admitted with diagnoses such as chest infection, subdural haematoma or lymphoma), others may have presented with complications of their underlying abdominal pathology leading to an incorrect initial diagnosis (sepsis, renal failure, anaemia, urinary tract infection, cardiac event) or were subject to an incorrect diagnosis at the time of their initial assessment. The latter usually led to admission under the care of a physician. This particularly included patients with a diagnosis of gastro-enteritis who were subsequently found to have surgical pathology to explain their symptoms. Thus a total of 274 patients died following surgery on an acute abdomen (Table 7.2.1).

**Table 7.2.1 Operation undertaken**

| Operation undertaken | n |
|---|---|
| Upper gastrointestinal surgery | 38 |
| Small/Large bowel surgery | 157 |
| Appendicectomy/hernia repair with abdominal surgery ± bowel resection | 25 |
| Aneurysm repair | 42 |
| Miscellaneous | 12 |
| **Total** | **274** |

## Initial assessment and decision making

Assessment after arrival at hospital appears to have been timely with the majority of patients (149/225) who underwent abdominal surgery reviewed within two hours (Figure 7.2.1).

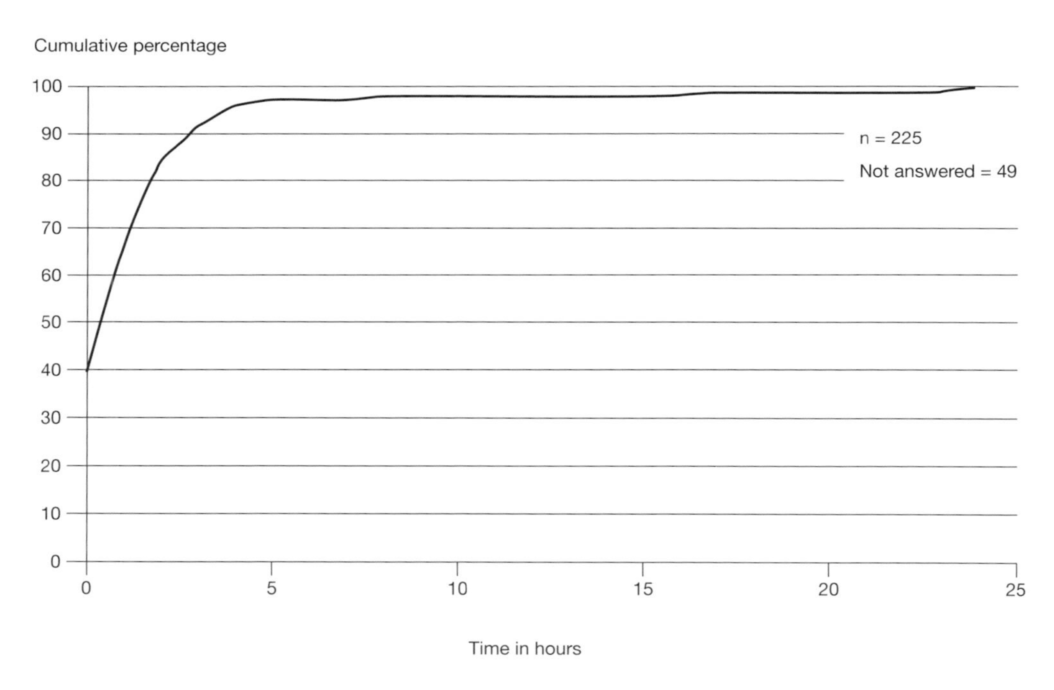


**Figure 7.2.1. Time between arrival and review**

For the majority of patients the initial assessment occurred in the emergency department or an assessment unit (Table 7.2.2) and was undertaken by a doctor in their early years of training (Figure 7.2.2) in either surgery or emergency medicine (Table 7.2.3).

**Table 7.2.2 Location of initial assessment**

| Location of initial assessment | n | % |
|---|---|---|
| Emergency department | 165 | 60.7 |
| Assessment unit | 81 | 29.8 |
| General ward | 8 | 2.9 |
| Specialist ward | 12 | 4.4 |
| Level 3 | 2 | <1 |
| Other | 4 | 1.5 |
| **Subtotal** | **272** | |
| Not answered | 2 | |
| **Total** | **274** | |

**Table 7.2.3 Specialty of the clinician undertaking the initial assessment**

| Specialty undertaking the initial assessment | n | % |
|---|---|---|
| General surgery | 105 | 43.4 |
| A&E | 68 | 28.1 |
| General medicine | 43 | 17.8 |
| Vascular surgery | 12 | 5.0 |
| Colorectal surgery | 5 | 2.1 |
| Geriatric medicine | 5 | 2.1 |
| Gastroenterology | 2 | <1 |
| Hepatobillary & Pancreatic surgery | 1 | <1 |
| Upper GI surgery | 1 | <1 |
| **Subtotal** | **242** | |
| Not answered | 32 | |
| **Total** | **274** | |

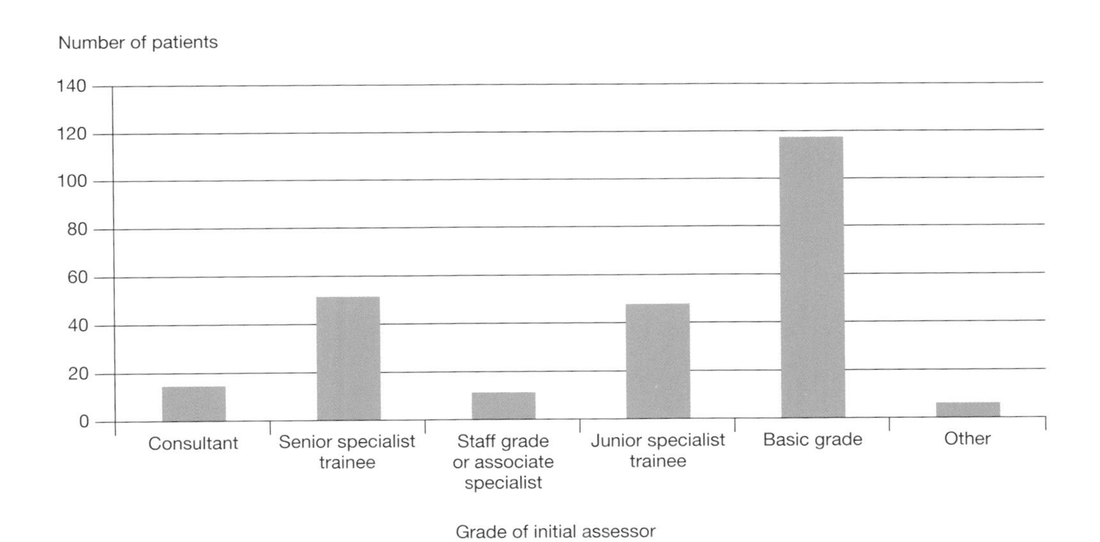


**Figure 7.2.2. Grade of clinician undertaking the initial assessment**

Following admission from the place of assessment a higher proportion of patients were initially assessed by a consultant or senior trainee when admitted under a surgeon (64%) rather than a physician (41%) (Table 7.2.4). Similarly it was more than twice as likely that initial assessment was undertaken by a basic grade doctor if the patient was admitted under the care of a physician. These differences had the potential to delay implementation of appropriate therapy, particularly when patients were admitted to a medical ward erroneously.

## Diagnosis and decision to operate

In most instances the diagnosis was made by a consultant (Table 7.2.6) who was undertaking the dedicated management of surgical emergencies rather than being committed to other clinical activities (Table 7.2.7). Thus, based on data derived from the surgical questionnaire, 237 of the surgeons were only responsible for the care of emergencies and/or in-patients when they made the diagnosis for patients included in this study.

**Table 7.2.4 Grade and specialty of the initial assessor following admission**

| | Surgery | Medicine | Subtotal | Not answered | Total |
|---|---|---|---|---|---|
| | n | n | n | n | n |
| Consultant | 55 | 13 | **68** | 2 | **70** |
| Senior specialist trainee | 62 | 13 | **75** | 9 | **84** |
| Staff grade or associate specialist | 10 | 2 | **12** | 1 | **13** |
| Junior specialist trainee | 26 | 12 | **38** | 2 | **40** |
| Basic grade | 29 | 23 | **52** | 9 | **61** |
| Other | 1 | 0 | **1** | 0 | **1** |
| **Subtotal** | **183** | **63** | **246** | **23** | **269** |
| Not answered | 1 | 4 | **5** | 0 | **5** |
| **Total** | **184** | **67** | **251** | **23** | **274** |

For the majority of patients the Advisors were of the opinion that clinicians provided a timely assessment of these patients and that this was undertaken by doctors of an appropriate level of expertise (Table 7.2.5).

**Table 7.2.5 Appropriateness of the time, grade and specialty of the initial assessment – Advisors' opinion**

| Appropriateness of initial assessment | n | % |
|---|---|---|
| Yes | 164 | 93.7 |
| No | 11 | 6.3 |
| **Subtotal** | **175** | |
| Unable to answer | 20 | |
| **Total** | **195** | |

**Table 7.2.6 Grade of the clinician making the diagnosis**

| Grade of clinician making the diagnosis | n | % |
|---|---|---|
| Consultant | 166 | 61.5 |
| Senior specialist trainee | 64 | 23.7 |
| Staff grade or associate specialist | 10 | 3.7 |
| Junior specialist trainee | 18 | 6.7 |
| Basic grade | 11 | 4.1 |
| Other | 1 | <1 |
| **Subtotal** | **270** | |
| Not answered | 4 | |
| **Total** | **274** | |

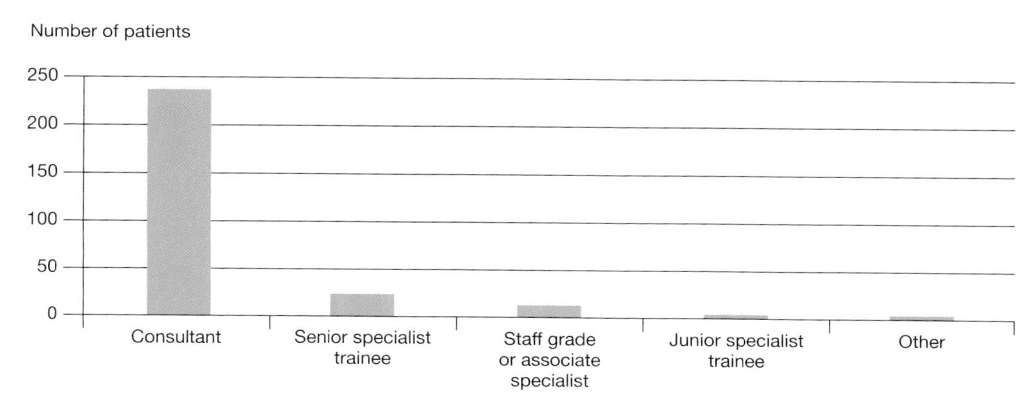


**Figure 7.2.3. Grade of the most senior clinician proposing the operation**

**Table 7.2.7 Other duties of the clinician making the diagnosis beyond being on call**

| Additional responsibilities | n* |
|---|---|
| Care of emergency admissions | 190 |
| Outpatient clinic | 27 |
| Inpatient ward care | 47 |
| Elective and diagnostic intervention | 17 |
| Elective operating list | 15 |
| Other | 6 |

** answers may be multiple*

In an overwhelming number of cases a consultant or senior trainee made the decision to proceed to abdominal surgery (Figure 7.2.3).

## The patients

Because of the age, comorbidities and the nature of the underlying pathology the health status (ASA grade) of this cohort at the time of admission was generally poor. Of more concern however was the deterioration in ASA grade between admission and the subsequent surgery. Figure 7.2.4 shows the ASA grade at operation for each ASA grade on admission. Thus, 6 ASA 2 patients deteriorated to ASA 3, 5 to ASA 4 and 2 to ASA 5 by the time of surgery. Similarly, although 7 ASA 3 patients improved to ASA 2, 33 deteriorated to ASA 4 and 9 to ASA 5. Three patients graded ASA 4 on admission improved to ASA 2, and 1 to ASA 3 although 5 deteriorated to ASA 5. Finally 2 patients admitted with ASA 5 improved to ASA 3 (1) or 4 (1).

This data indicates that the predominant trend was for ASA grade to worsen rather than improve between admission and surgery. This implies that resuscitation had a minimal impact on improving health status. It is important to remember however these ASA grades were gathered retrospectively by the surgeon completing the questionnaire.

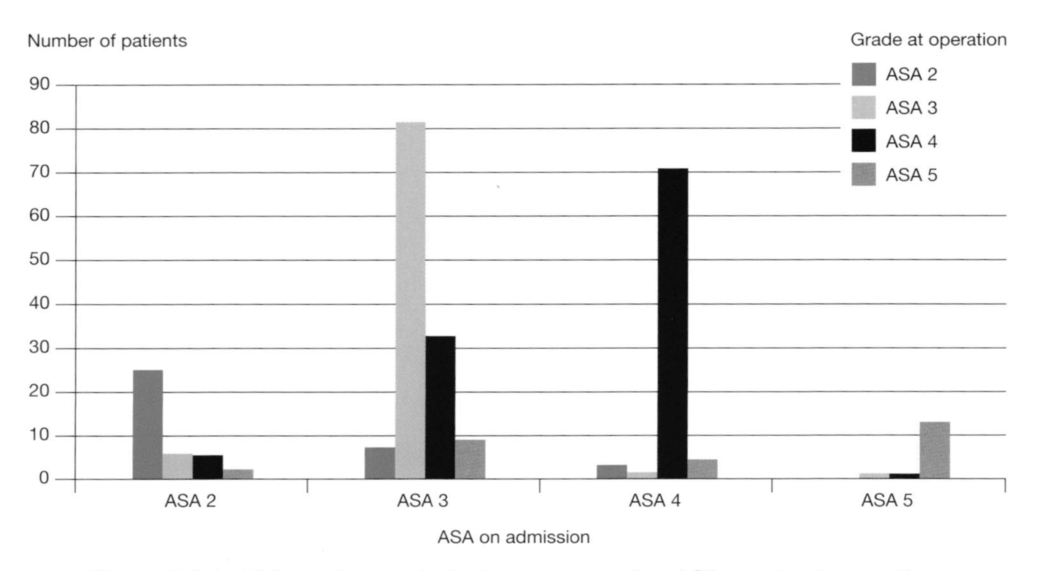


**Figure 7.2.4. ASA grade on admission compared to ASA grade at operation**

There are a number of scenarios that might explain the deterioration in ASA grade between admission and surgery. Clearly it could be related to the severity of the underlying pathology. Alternative causes include a delay between the decision to operate and performing surgery and a failure to undertake adequate pre-operative resuscitation.

Whilst it is not possible to attribute the deterioration in ASA grade to one of these particular causes there was evidence to suggest that a delay in performing surgery may have contributed to some deaths. Thus Table 7.2.8 confirms that the reporting surgeons considered that there had been a delay in performing abdominal surgery in 82 of these patients with 13 waiting 5 days or more. Figure 7.2.5 indicates the extent of these delays.

There are no data which explain why these delays occurred although the Advisors considered that surgery was not performed in a timely manner in 22% of patients (Table 7.2.9). This is disappointing given that the overwhelming majority of patients were considered to require either immediate or urgent surgery by the consultants responsible for their care (Figure 7.2.6).

**Table 7.2.8 Delays noted between admission and operation**

| Delays between admission and operation | n | % |
|---|---|---|
| Yes | 82 | 30.6 |
| No | 181 | 67.5 |
| Unknown | 5 | 1.9 |
| **Subtotal** | **268** | |
| Not answered | 6 | |
| **Total** | **274** | |

**Table 7.2.9 Timeliness of the operation performed – Advisors' opinion**

| Operation timely | n | % |
|---|---|---|
| Yes | 149 | 78.4 |
| No | 41 | 21.6 |
| **Subtotal** | **190** | |
| Unable to answer | 4 | |
| Not answered | 1 | |
| **Total** | **195** | |

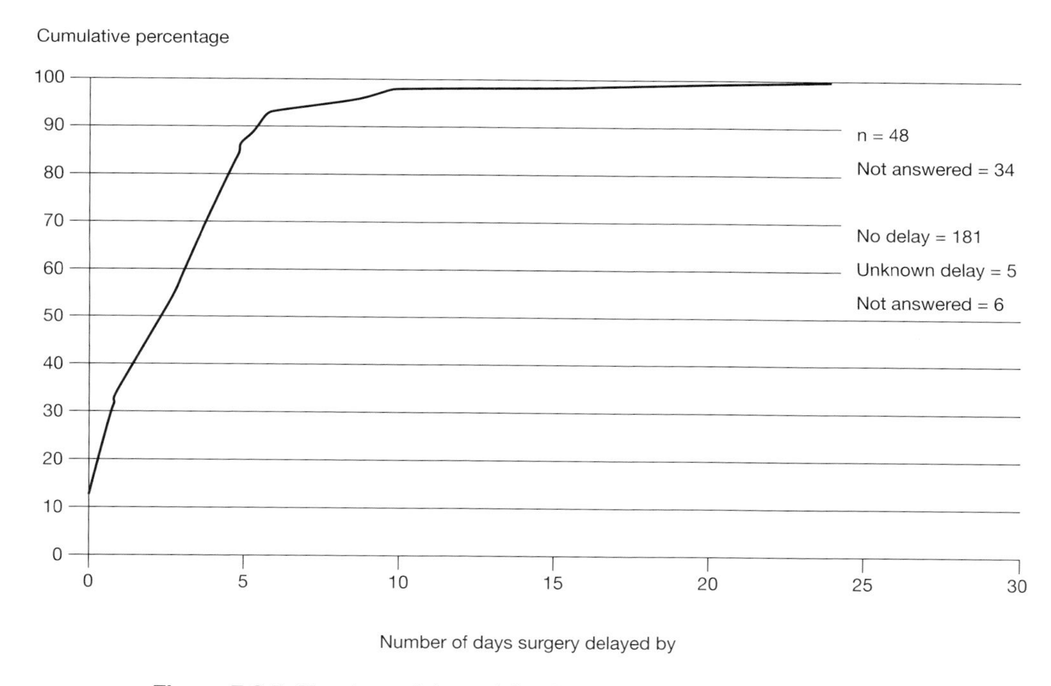


**Figure 7.2.5. Number of days delay between surgery and operation**

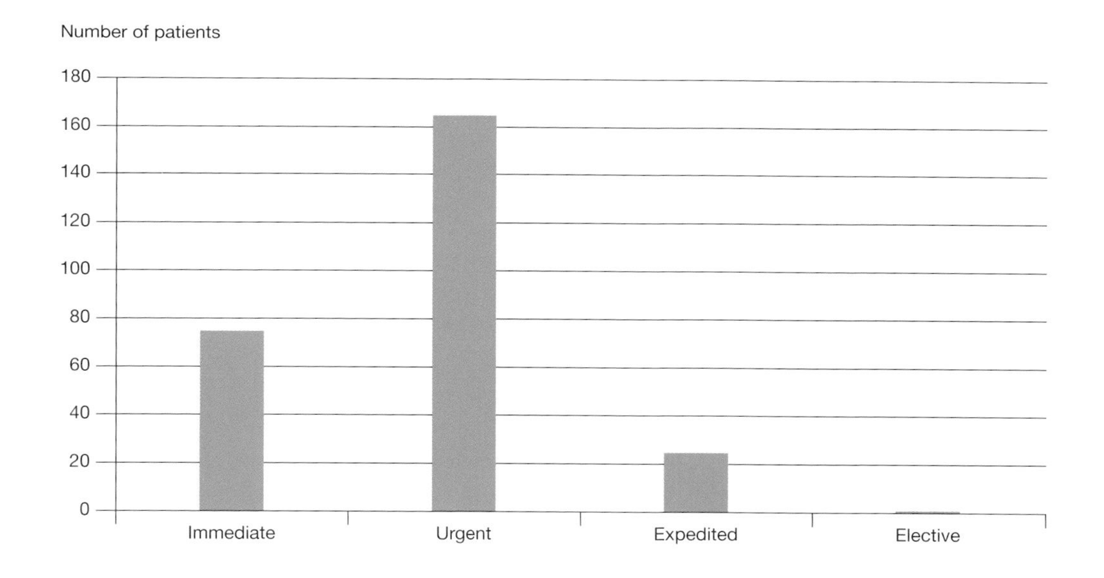


**Figure 7.2.6. Classification of the procedure**

## Surgery

Although a decision was made to undertake surgery in all of these patients this was not always performed with the expectation of patient survival (Table 7.2.10). This raises the issue highlighted in the introduction to this chapter of subjecting elderly patients with ASA scores of 4 or 5 to intervention. Data from this report cannot answer this question. This would require a prospective audit of such patients with the aim of developing a robust method of risk assessment.

**Table 7.2.10 Expectation of survival**

| Expectation to survive | n | % |
|---|---|---|
| Yes | 117 | 43.5 |
| No | 43 | 16.0 |
| Unknown | 109 | 40.5 |
| **Subtotal** | **269** | |
| Not answered | 5 | |
| **Total** | **274** | |

Despite the sometimes gloomy predictions about survival the majority of these operations were performed in anticipation of achieving cure for the underlying pathology (Table 7.2.11) this indicating most patients died from conditions which were thought by their surgeons, even in retrospect, to be survivable.

**Table 7.2.11 Operative intent**

| Operative intent | n | % |
|---|---|---|
| Diagnostic | 17 | 6.3 |
| Diagnostic and curative | 22 | 8.2 |
| Diagnostic and curative and palliative | 1 | <1 |
| Diagnostic and palliative | 9 | 3.4 |
| Curative | 180 | 67.2 |
| Palliative | 39 | 14.6 |
| **Subtotal** | **268** | |
| Not answered | 6 | |
| **Total** | **274** | |

For most of these operations the senior surgeon present at the start of surgery was either a consultant or a senior trainee (246/271) (Figure 7.2.7). Additional data that is not presented here confirms that suitable surgical assistants were available in the operating theatre despite the possible influence of European Working Time Directive (EWTD) and shift work.

In 87/274 operations the surgeon performing the operation was not a consultant. Where this was the case the level of supervision by the responsible consultant was as shown in Table 7.2.12.

**Table 7.2.12 Level of supervision if the primary operator was not a consultant**

| Level of supervision | n |
|---|---|
| Supervised scrubbed | 17 |
| Unsupervised in theatre | 16 |
| Unsupervised in hospital | 33 |
| Other | 14 |
| **Subtotal** | **80** |
| Not answered | 7 |
| **Total** | **87** |

On the basis of this information the Advisors were of the opinion that the level of supervision was inadequate in almost a third of those cases in which it could be assessed (Table 7.2.13). For these 13 operations adequate documentation was available for 11 and showed that surgery was performed by an unsupervised trainee in all instances. Unfortunately the data was insufficient to allow a definitive view for the remainder of operations. In 128 cases the operation was carried out by a consultant, and in 3 cases the grade of operating surgeon was not given.

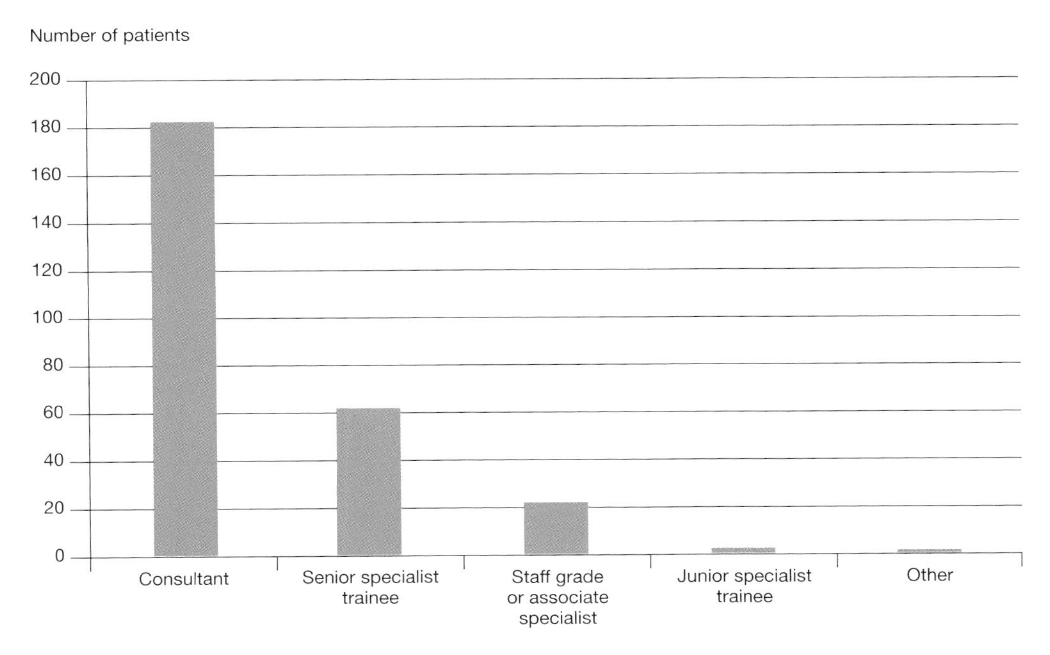


**Figure 7.2.7. Grade of the most senior operating surgeon?**

**Table 7.2.13 Adequacy of supervision if the surgeon was not a consultant – Advisors' opinion**

| Adequate supervision | n |
|---|---|
| Yes | 19 |
| No | 13 |
| **Subtotal** | **32** |
| Unable to answer | 22 |
| Not answered | 10 |
| **Total** | **64** |

**Table 7.2.14 Evidence that junior staff did not seek appropriate advice when necessary – Advisors' opinion**

| Junior staff did not seek advice as necessary | n | % |
|---|---|---|
| Yes | 39 | 21.0 |
| No | 147 | 79.0 |
| **Subtotal** | **186** | |
| Unable to answer | 9 | |
| **Total** | **195** | |

In the same vein, although not specifically related to the operation, the Advisors were of the opinion that on many occasions non-consultant surgical and anaesthetic staff did not seek appropriate advice from a consultant when this would have been appropriate (Table 7.2.14).

The following case study presents some of the issues raised so far in this chapter.

**Case Study 24**

An independent patient attended the Emergency Department with vomiting, one loose stool, and dehydration. An abdominal X-ray was performed, but the dilated small bowel was not recognised by a basic trainee and no senior review was undertaken. The patient was admitted under MCOP with presumed gastroenteritis and clerked by an Foundation Year 2 doctor who suspected an obstructed right groin hernia. This was not confirmed until review by an MCOP registrar three days later when surgical referral was made and femoral hernia repair and laparotomy with small bowel resection were performed by an inexperienced registrar. This was complicated by an anasotomotic leak and after a further delay laparotomy was undertaken for faecal peritonitis. The patient died 48 hours later. The death was not reported to the coroner.

*Advisors felt that more senior initial assessment both in the Emergency Department and on the medical ward would have led to the correct diagnosis and early surgery. Further, an inexperienced registrar did not seek advice and thus was not supervised during the first operation.*

## Outcomes in patients not considered to have acute abdominal pathology on admission

As indicated above there were 35 patients who did not have a diagnosis of an acute abdomen on admission, but who went on to undergo an abdominal procedure.

Of these only 3 were admitted with a diagnosis that might have been considered entirely remote or unrelated to the final diagnosis. That this was not appreciated at the time of the initial assessment might have been related to the seniority of the clinician performing this; only 8/35 patients were initially assessed by a consultant or senior trainee (Table 7.2.15). This may be particularly relevant given that these patients are likely to have provided a diagnostic challenge.

**Table 7.2.15 Grade of clinician undertaking the initial assessment on arrival**

| Grade | n |
|---|---|
| Consultant | 1 |
| Senior specialist trainee | 7 |
| Staff grade or associate specialist | 2 |
| Junior specialist trainee | 3 |
| Basic grade | 18 |
| Other | 1 |
| Not answered | 3 |
| **Total** | **35** |

A further indication of the possible inadequacy of the initial assessment is reflected by the specialty under which the patients were admitted. Thus only 7 patients were admitted under the care of an abdominal surgeon and 3 under another surgical specialty. Twenty three patients were admitted under the care of a physician and in one case the admitting specialty was not given. Whilst this had little impact on the delay to first consultant review (Table 7.2.16) it may have been important in respect of the timeliness with which surgery was performed (Table 7.2.17). Where an opinion could be given the Advisors considered that surgery was not performed in a timely manner in 8/21 of these 35 patients compared to 35/172 for all of the other patients undergoing abdominal surgery.

**Table 7.2.16 Evidence of a delay in consultant review – Advisors' opinion**

| Delay in consultant review | Patients not initially admitted with a diagnosis of an acute abdomen (n) | Patient admitted with a diagnosis of an acute abdomen (n) |
|---|---|---|
| Yes | 5 | 23 |
| No | 15 | 114 |
| **Subtotal** | **20** | **137** |
| Unable to answer | 3 | 37 |
| Not answered | 0 | 1 |
| **Total** | **23** | **175** |

**Table 7.2.17 Timeliness of the surgery undertaken – Advisors' opinion**

| Surgery carried out in a timely manner | Patients not initially admitted with a diagnosis of an acute abdomen (n) | Patient admitted with a diagnosis of an acute abdomen (n) |
|---|---|---|
| Yes | 13 | 137 |
| No | 8 | 35 |
| **Subtotal** | **21** | **172** |
| Unable to answer | 2 | 3 |
| Not answered | 0 | 1 |
| **Total** | **23** | **175** |

In summary there was a subgroup of patients who presented with apparently non-specific symptoms or signs that were often consistent with sepsis or cardiovascular instability. That they had underlying abdominal pathology was not recognised at their initial assessment and thus they were usually admitted under the care of a physician. These patients suffered delays prior to undergoing abdominal surgery.

## Anaesthetic provision

For patients undergoing abdominal surgery the level of anaesthetic cover in relation to the ASA grade at operation is shown in Table 7.2.18. Overall, 132/178 of anaesthetics were delivered by a consultant, irrespective of the ASA grade. Somewhat disappointingly this proportion did not increase dramatically in patient's assigned ASA grades 4 or 5 where the most senior anaesthetist was a trainee or staff grade in 19/98 of cases.

**Table 7.2.18 Grade of most senior anaesthetist providing the anaesthetic by ASA prior to surgery**

| Grade of most senior anaesthetist (n) | ASA 2 | ASA 3 | ASA 4 | ASA 5 | Subtotal | Not answered | Total |
|---|---|---|---|---|---|---|---|
| Consultant | 17 | 36 | 62 | 17 | **132** | 7 | **139** |
| Senior specialist trainee | 2 | 13 | 9 | 1 | **25** | 0 | **25** |
| Staff grade or associate specialist | 2 | 4 | 6 | 1 | **13** | 0 | **13** |
| Junior specialist trainee | 2 | 3 | 0 | 1 | **6** | 0 | **15** |
| Basic grade | 0 | 0 | 1 | 0 | 1 | 0 | **6** |
| Other | 0 | 1 | 0 | 0 | 1 | 0 | **1** |
| **Subtotal** | **23** | **57** | **78** | **20** | **178** | **7** | **185** |
| Not answered | 0 | 0 | 1 | 0 | **1** | 0 | **1** |
| **Total** | **23** | **57** | **79** | **20** | **179** | **7** | **186** |

**ASA Prior to surgery (n)**

## Peri-operative care

***Prophylaxis for thromboembolic disease***

Implementation of appropriate prophylaxis for thromboembolic disease remains an important issue despite having been highlighted in previous NCEPOD reports[8] and the relatively recent publication of NICE guidelines for surgical patients.[9] Even though this cohort of patients was elderly and all were proceeding to abdominal surgery the responsible surgeon did not always consider that they were at risk of venous thrombosis (Table 7.2.19).

**Table 7.2.19 Risk factors for venous thrombosis**

| Risk factors for venous thrombosis | n | % |
|---|---|---|
| No patient related risk factors | 32 | 12.7 |
| One or more patient related risk factors | 219 | 87.3 |
| **Subtotal** | **251** | |
| Not answered | 23 | |
| **Total** | **274** | |

In the opinion of the Advisors assessment was inadequate in many of these patients (Table 7.2.20).

**Table 7.2.20 Appropriateness of the risk assessed for thrombotic complications – Advisors' opinion**

| Appropriate assessment for thrombotic complications | n | % |
|---|---|---|
| Yes | 112 | 82.4 |
| No | 24 | 17.6 |
| **Subtotal** | **136** | |
| Unable to answer | 54 | |
| Not answered | 5 | |
| **Total** | **195** | |

Where prophylaxis was prescribed low molecular weight heparin (162/219) and graduated compression stockings (128/219) were most frequently used, often in combination. This is consistent with the NICE guidelines.

***Peri-operative antibiotics***

These were prescribed for the majority of patients and there did not seem to be any issues relating to this aspect of care.

## Global patient assessment

***Nutrition***

A formal nutritional assessment was only performed in a minority of patients (Table 7.2.21). This is likely to have had an adverse impact in those patients who died following a protracted period of post operative care. A more detailed discussion about the nutritional requirements of elderly surgical patients is included in Chapter 4. Nevertheless it is clear that this aspect of management should be improved.

**Table 7.2.21 Formal nutritional assessment undertaken on admission**

| Nutritional assessment undertaken | n | % |
|---|---|---|
| Yes | 32 | 12.0 |
| No | 195 | 73.0 |
| Unknown | 40 | 15.0 |
| **Subtotal** | **267** | |
| Not answered | 7 | |
| **Total** | **274** | |

***Skin viability***

It also appears that assessment of skin viability, and presumably the implementation of appropriate measures to prevent pressure ulcers and their complications were not widely adopted in this cohort of critically ill patients

(Table 7.2.22). The combination of poor nutrition, limited mobility, sepsis and the increased prevalence of vascular disease in these patients puts them at high risk.

**Table 7.2.22 Assessment of skin viability**

| Assessment of skin viability | n | % |
|---|---|---|
| Yes | 89 | 35.9 |
| No | 64 | 25.8 |
| Unknown | 95 | 38.3 |
| **Subtotal** | **248** | |
| Not answered | 26 | |
| **Total** | **274** | |

## Medicine for the Care of Older People (MCOP)

In most of the surgical units where these operations were performed there was no formal arrangement for regular input from MCOP. Even where this occurred it generally comprised an on-call or referral service with little evidence of the ability to deliver co-ordinated care. Given this, it is not surprising that few of the patients were ever reviewed by the MCOP team during their admission. This data is summarised in Tables 7.2.23, 7.2.24 and 7.2.25.

**Table 7.2.23 Formal regular input from MCOP to the surgical team**

| Regular input from MCOP to the surgical team | n | % |
|---|---|---|
| Yes | 81 | 30.6 |
| No | 157 | 59.2 |
| Unknown | 27 | 10.2 |
| **Subtotal** | **265** | |
| Not answered | 9 | |
| **Total** | **274** | |

**Table 7.2.24 Degree of formal MCOP input**

| What does any input from MCOP constitute | n* |
|---|---|
| Weekly ward round | 10 |
| Input into guidelines and policies | 7 |
| On call service only/referral service | 68 |
| Other | 7 |

*answers may be multiple*

**Table 7.2.25 Review by an MCOP consultant if not admitted under MCOP**

| Reviews by MCOP consultant | n | % |
|---|---|---|
| Yes | 15 | 6.7 |
| No | 195 | 86.7 |
| Unknown | 15 | 6.7 |
| **Subtotal** | **225** | |
| Not answered | 31 | |
| **Total** | **256** | |

Eight patients with an acute abdomen were admitted under MCOP. In 10 cases the admitting specialty was not recorded in the surgical questionnaire.

These data do not compare favourably with that for patients undergoing surgery for fractured neck of femur (42.5%) included in this study (see Chapter 7.1).

This level of medical input for patients with an acute abdomen with a high incidence of medical comorbidities is unsatisfactory and requires addressing as a matter of urgency.

## Key findings

Initial assessment of patients, following arrival in the hospital was timely in this group (149/225 cases reviewed within 2 hours of arrival).

There was a high level of consultant surgeon involvement in both making the diagnosis and more particularly in the decision to perform surgery for patients included in this study.

Following admission patients in this population were less likely to be assessed by a consultant if they were admitted to a medical specialty.

Advisors judged the operation not to be performed in a timely manner in 41/190 cases in this group.

Junior staff failed to seek advice about patient management or surgery in 39/186 of patients requiring abdominal surgery.

Input from MCOP was infrequent and markedly less than in patients admitted with a fractured neck of femur.

Recognition of the need for thromboprophylaxis in this group of patients remains sub-optimal. Furthermore, routine assessment of their nutritional requirements and skin viability were poor.

Patients presenting with non-specific abdominal symptoms or signs of sepsis but who subsequently required abdominal surgery were usually admitted under the care of a physician. This may have reduced awareness of the underlying surgical pathology and was associated with greater delays in performing surgery.

## Recommendations

Greater vigilance is required when elderly patients with non-specific abdominal symptoms and signs (diarrhoea, vomiting, constipation, urinary tract infection) present to the Emergency Department. Such patients should be assessed by a doctor with sufficient experience and training to exclude significant surgical pathology. (Trusts, Clinical Directors)

The elderly should receive no different level of care from other patients. As NCEPOD has previously recommended[10] when admitted to a medical ward consultant review should occur within 12 hours. (Consultants)

Clear protocols for the post operative management of elderly patients undergoing abdominal surgery should be developed which include where appropriate routine review by a MCOP consultant and nutritional assessment. (Clinical Directors)

A robust method of risk assessment for elderly patients presenting with an acute intra-abdominal catastrophe should be developed.

Trusts should audit delays in proceeding to surgery in patients requiring emergency or urgent abdominal surgery and implement appropriate mechanisms to reduce these. (Trusts, Clinical Directors)

***References***


1. Madsen MR. Laparotomy in patients aged 80 years and older. A prospective analysis of morbidity during 1 year in the county of Ringkobing. *Ugeskrift for Laeger*; 1993, 155(37), 2878-81

2. Ford PNR, Thomas I et al. Determinants of outcome in critically ill octogenarians after surgery: an observational study. *British Journal of Anaesthesia*; 2007; 99(6), 824 - 829

3. Louis DJ, Hsu A, et al.Morbidity and mortality in octogenarians and older undergoing major intestinal surgery. *Disease of the Colon & Rectum;* 2009, 52, 59 - 63

4. Cook TM & Day CJE. Hospital mortality after urgent and emergency laparotomy in patients aged 65 yr and over. Risk and prediction of risk using multiple logistic regression analysis. *British Journal of Anaesthesia.* 1998; 80, 776 - 781

5. Monod-Broca P. Mortality in emergency abdominal surgery. 304 cases. A plea for better clinical practice. *Annales de Gastroenterologie et d Hepatologie*; 1990, 26(4), 184 - 6

6. Church, JM. Laparotomy for acute colorectal conditions in moribund patients: is it worthwhile? *Diseases of the Colon & Rectum*; 2005, 48(6), 1147 - 52

7. Toulson Davisson Correia MI, Costa Fonseca P, & Machado Cruz GA. Perioperative nutritional management of patients undergoing laparotomy. *Nutricion Hospitalaria*; 2009, 24(4), 479 - 84

8. National Confidential Enquiry into Patient Outcome and Death. *Caring to the end?* 2009. NCEPOD, London

9. National Institute for Health and Clinical Excellence. *Venous Thromboembolism – reducing the risk*. 2010. National Institute for Health and Clinical Excellence

10. National Confidential Enquiry into Patient Outcome and Death. Emergency admissions: *A journey in the right direction?*. 2007. NCEPOD, London.

# 8 - Pathology

## Reporting deaths to coroners

Under the current coronial legislation[1] and regulations[2], deaths following a surgical procedure are usually reported to a coroner. The coroner makes investigations into the circumstances of the death, to determine whether:

- The case comes into the category of suspected 'violent or unnatural' cause of death, or the cause of death is 'unknown'[1]
- The clinicians and/or the family have any concerns about the circumstances of death

...and thus make a decision whether or not to commission an autopsy under s19 (usually) or s20 of the Coroner Act 1988, the prime purpose of the autopsy being to determine whether an inquest is necessary into the case.[3] Peri-operative deaths, per se, are not statutorily reportable to coroners, although most jurisdictions issue a local instruction to do so.

If the autopsy result is not an 'unnatural' cause of death, there is no legal requirement to hold an inquest, although many such do take place.[4]

In this study population, of the three-quarters of cases where information was complete, 62% (674/1084) of the deaths were reported to coroners and 14.9% (162/1084) were not (Table 8.1); and the coroners accepted 22% (145/643) for further autopsy examination. It was unknown in 100 cases whether the coroner accepted the case and not answered in 31 cases.

**Table 8.1 Reporting to a coroner**

| Case reported to coroner | n | % |
|---|---|---|
| Yes | 674 | 62.2 |
| No | 162 | 14.9 |
| Unknown | 248 | 22.9 |
| **Subtotal** | **1084** | |
| Not answered | 36 | |
| **Total** | **1120** | |

Current overall national rates of reporting to, and acceptance by, coroners (all causes of death – in hospital and community) are both 46%[4], and these have not changed significantly for 2 years. The high reporting rate here (62%) reflects the encouragement to report all peri-operative deaths. The lower than average rate of accepting cases for autopsy probably reflects the more complete information derived from being in hospital, investigated, and operated upon, and may also reflect the age of the patient cohort.

## Consented autopsies

If the coroner does not require further investigations, and a medical certificate of cause of death (MCCD) is written by a clinician (and is a 'natural' cause of death), then the clinicians involved can ask the family for permission to undertake an autopsy examination, to determine more precisely what happened. In this study, the great majority of deaths were not so pursued (834), with only 14 requests for autopsy indicated, and at least 573 responses stated 'no request for autopsy'. In 272 it was not answered whether a hospital autopsy was requested.

Sadly, this is congruent with current trends, where <5% of deaths among babies outside the perinatal period are followed by a consented, hospital autopsy.[4] For complex reasons, the UK trend is for hospital clinicians not to be particularly interested in autopsy examination and for families often to refuse if so requested. In rare cases, families may request a private autopsy on a relative, including a second autopsy if there has already been a coronial examination, but we were not aware of any such autopsies among this study's cases.

### Autopsy feedback to clinicians

Of the 159 case autopsies done (145 coronial + 14 requested), only 57% (78/136) of the responding surgeons stated that they had received a copy of the autopsy report. No autopsy report was received in 41 cases, it was unknown in 17, and not answered in 23. Whilst biased by some absent responses, this is not an encouraging statistic, and is no improvement on the data in previous NCEPOD reports. The coronial system, and its pathologists, need to inform clinicians about their patients' outcomes.

### Autopsy quality

This report has not investigated the quality of autopsy, the topic having been considered fully in earlier NCEPOD reports.[3] Moreover, there should be significant changes to the investigation and certification of death with the implementation, from 2012, of the Coroner and Justice Act 2009.[5]

Further, the report is not presenting details of the overall causes of death in the study population; they were very heterogeneous, and biased by the nature of case selection.

### Information from autopsies

The NCEPOD Advisors were asked to state if an autopsy, coronial or hospital, delivered any unexpected findings. In 15 cases there were, the three most common scenarios being ischaemic bowel, leaks in the bowel, and pulmonary thromboembolism.

### Medical certificates of cause of death

The NCEPOD assessors were asked to comment on the accuracy of the medical certificates of cause of death as completed by clinicians. The great majority (85%, 370/439) were found to be satisfactory (i.e. congruent with known clinical circumstances of the death), but in 69 cases they were not; furthermore, in 381 cases the Advisors were unable to answers this. For 62 of these, the assessors provided alternative MCCD or a comment; these comments are highlighted in Table 8.2. These data shed light on the known problems in ensuring clinicians both report the right cases to coroners, and complete death certificates more acurately - sadly they are an unpaid activity, often regarded as a chore, ill-taught in medical school and postgraduate training, and un-audited in clinical practice.[6,7,8]

**Table 8.2 The main issues highlighted by the assessors concerning appropriate of medical certificates of causes of death**

| Main issues concerning the appropriate MCCD | n |
|---|---|
| Would have reported the case to a coroner | 6 |
| No mention of the surgery in the cause of death sequence | 11 |
| Wrong cause of death | 9 |
| Omission of an healthcare associated infection (HCAI) in the MCCD | 2 |
| Omission of dementia as a significant contribution | 2 |
| Wrong structure/order of the MCCD, but the correct disease | 2 |

The unmentioned Health Care Associated Infections (HCAI) were both *Clostridium difficile* colitis. Not mentioning the surgical procedure is unhelpful, since the Office for National Statistics tries to correlate diseases and outcomes, and it is a standard recommendation from both the WHO and the ONS that surgery for relevant terminal disease must be included in the MCCD.

The 'wrong' causes of death are – of course – the opinion of the assessors who have read part or all of the available clinical records. However, over- and under-diagnosis of cancer are included here, as are omitted pulmonary embolism and gastro-intestinal bleeding, and under-diagnosis of systemic sepsis.

**Final comment on Old Age and MCCDs.**

Reviewing the hundreds of medical certificates of cause of death across the study, it is striking how uncommonly 'Old Age' (19), 'Dementia' (19) and 'Frailty' (5) were mentioned. Yet the message coming across from the clinical analyses is how frail these elderly patients were, how important dementia was in communication and prognostication, and how many of the pathologies encountered are really just manifestations of age-related, irreversible organ degeneration.

Clinicians still think in terms of specific physical diseases, naturally, but perhaps are ignoring more important contributions towards these patients' deaths. Are we doing our ageing population, and collectively ourselves, a disservice if we fail to give appropriate acknowledgement to the more generic issues, when we do not consider them worthy of mention in the final statement written on the metaphorical tombstone?

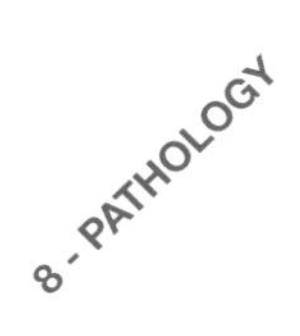


### *References*


1. Coroner Act. 1998. Crown Copyright

2. Coroners Rules. 1984. Crown Copyright

3. National Confidential Enquiry into Patient Outcome and Death. *The Coroners Autopsy: Do we deserve better?* 2006. NCEPOD, London

4. Ministry of Justice. Statistics on deaths reported to coroners. England and Wales, 2009. *Ministry of Justice Statistics Bulletin.* 2010. Crown Copyright.

5. Coroners and Justice Act. 2009. Crown Copyright

6. Swift B, West K. Death certification: an audit of practice entering the 21st century. J Clin Pathol 2005, 55:275-279

7. Gladwin J and Clarke A. Information Management Strategies and Death Certification in the UK. Health Informatics Journal 2003 9: 283 http://jhi.sagepub.com/content/9/4/283.full.pdf+html

8. Devis T, Rooney C. Death certification and the epidemiologist. Health Statistics Quarterly 01, Spring 1999, 21-32

# Appendicies

## Appendix 1

### Principal recommendations from *Adding Insult to Injury*

All patients admitted as an emergency, regardless of specialty, should have their electrolytes checked routinely on admission and appropriately thereafter. This will prevent the insidious and unrecognised onset of AKI. (Clinical Directors and Medical Directors)

Predictable and avoidable AKI should never occur. For those in-patients who develop AKI there should be both a robust assessment of contributory risk factors and an awareness of the possible complications that may arise. (Clinical Directors and Medical Directors)

All acute admissions should receive adequate senior reviews (with a consultant review within 12 hours of admission as previously recommended by NCEPOD). (Clinical Directors and Medical Directors)

NCEPOD recommends that the guidance for recognising the acutely ill patient (NICE CG 50) is disseminated and implemented. In particular all acute patients should have admission physiological observations performed and a written physiological monitoring plan made, taking into account the degree of illness and risk of deterioration. (Clinical Directors and Medical Directors)

There should be sufficient critical care and renal beds to allow rapid step up in care if appropriate. (Department of Health)

All level 3 units should have the ability to deliver renal replacement therapy; and where appropriate these patients should receive clinical input from a nephrologist. (Clinical Directors and Medical Directors)

All acute admitting hospitals should have access to either onsite nephrologists or a dedicated nephrology service within reasonable distance of the admitting hospital. (Clinical Directors and Medical Directors)

All acute admitting hospitals should have access to a renal ultrasound scanning service 24 hours a day including the weekends and the ability to provide emergency relief of renal obstruction. (Clinical Directors and Medical Directors)

# Appendix 2

## Glossary

| | |
|---|---|
| AF | Atrial Fibrilation |
| APS | Acute Pain Service |
| ASA | American Society of Anaesthesiologists score |
| BMI | Body Mass Index |
| BOA | British Orthopaedic Association |
| COPD | Chronic Obstructive Pulmonary Disease |
| CT | Computerised Tomography |
| CVA | Cerebrovascular Accident |
| DGH | District General Hospital |
| DH | Department of Health |
| ED | Emergency Department |
| EDTA | Ethylenediaminetetraacetic acid |
| ELCP | End of Life Care Pathway |
| FBC | Full blood count |
| Fractured NOF | Fractured Neck of Femur |
| FY | Foundation Year |
| GCS | Glasgow Coma Scale |
| GI | Gastro Intestinal |
| GP | General Practitioner |
| Hb | Haemoglobin |
| HDU | High Dependency Unit |
| ICU | Intensive Care Unit |
| IHD | Ischaemic Heart Disease |
| LFT | Liver Function Test |
| MCCD | Medical Certificate of Cause of Death |
| MCOP | Medicine for the Care of Older People and Medicine for the Elderly |
| MDT | Multidisciplinary Team |
| MI | Myocardial Infarction |
| NICE | National Institute for Health and Clinical Excellence |
| NSAID | Non Steriodal Anti Inflamatory |
| NSF | National Service Framework |
| OPCS | Office of Population Censuses and Surveys |
| PACU | Post Anaesthetic Care Unit |
| PCA | Patient Controlled Analgesia |
| POCD | Post Operative Cognitive Dysfunction |
| QIPP | Quality, Innovation, Productivity and Prevention |
| RCoA | Royal College of Anaesthetists |
| RCP | Royal College of Physicians |
| RCS | Royal College of Surgeons |
| SAS | Staff Grade or Associate Specialist |
| SHO | Senior House Officer |
| SIGN | Scottish Intercollegiate Guidelines Network |
| SpR | Specialist Registrar |
| T&O | Trauma & Orthopaedics |
| TIA | Transient Ischaemic Attack |
| U&E | Urea and Electrolytes |
| VTE | Venous Thromboembolism |
| WHO | World Health Organisation |

# Appendix 3

## Corporate structure and role of NCEPOD

The National Confidential Enquiry into Patient Outcome and Death (NCEPOD) is an independent body to which a corporate commitment has been made by the Medical and Surgical Colleges, Associations and Faculties related to its area of activity. Each of these bodies nominates members on to NCEPOD's Steering Group.

***The role of NCEPOD***

The role of NCEPOD is to describe the gap between the care that should be delivered and what actually happens on the ground. In some ways it is a glorious anachronism: an exercise by the professions themselves to criticise the care that they deliver in the cause of improving the quality of the Service.

The process is simple but effective. We begin with an idea. Subjects can be suggested by anyone, but most come from the professional associations. It is measure of how deeply the medical profession are committed to the improvement of their service that they should be voluble and enthusiastic about having the care that they deliver assessed and criticised by their peers.

We have far more proposals than we can carry out and each year studies are chosen by competitive secret ballot of the NCEPOD Steering Group, after what is often a lively and partisan debate. In November 2007, when *Parenteral Nutrition* was chosen with *Surgery in the Elderly*, there were a further 12 disappointed studies.

Having gained Steering Group approval, the staff and Clinical Co-ordinators together with an expert group work up the study design so as to get the raw material that they think they will need to explore the quality of care. They identify a given group of cases and design the study and the questionnaires.

The NCEPOD Local Reporters – our precious eyes and ears in every Trust - are then asked to identify all the cases falling within that cohort. We then send all the Consultants responsible for those cases a questionnaire and elicit the key data that we need. We also ask the Trusts for copies of the notes.

Our staff then go through the notes laboriously anonymising them so that that the Advisors and Authors cannot identify the patient, the hospital or the staff involved. Inevitably from time to time a perspicacious Advisor will recognise a colleague's handwriting, or even a case from their own hospital: they are trusted to quietly replace it on the pile and draw another.

The Advisors are specialists in the areas of the study but they are emphatically not members of the expert group and play no part in the design of the study. They may have no prior connection with NCEPOD but wish to contribute to the over-riding aim of improving care in their specialty. They are trained, being put through dummy runs together with our Co-ordinators, so as to develop the necessary consistency of approach. Their assessment of the cases is done in our premises, in group meetings. Most cases will only be read by one Advisor who fills in a questionnaire, but they work together and discuss striking features as they come across them, so that the finished report and the vignettes do not represent idiosyncratic opinions. As you can see from our Acknowledgements they are a multidisciplinary group of distinguished professionals and the final report is compiled by the Co-ordinators and our staff from the material and the judgements made by them, for which we are deeply grateful.

***Steering Group as at 11th November 2010***

| | |
|---|---|
| Dr R Birks | Association of Anaesthetists of Great Britain and Ireland |
| Mr T Bates | Association of Surgeons of Great Britain & Ireland |
| Mr J Wardrope | College of Emergency Medicine |
| Dr S Bridgman | Faculty of Public Health Medicine |
| Professor R Mahajan | Royal College of Anaesthetists |
| Dr A Batchelor | Royal College of Anaesthetists |
| Dr B Ellis | Royal College of General Practitioners |
| Ms M McElligott | Royal College of Nursing |
| Dr T Falconer | Royal College of Obstetricians and Gynaecologists |
| Mrs M Wishart | Royal College of Ophthalmologists |
| Dr I Doughty | Royal College of Paediatrics and Child Health |
| Dr R Dowdle | Royal College of Physicians |
| Professor T Hendra | Royal College of Physicians |
| Dr M Clements | Royal College of Physicians |
| Dr S McPherson | Royal College of Radiologists |
| Mr B Rees | Royal College of Surgeons of England |
| Mr M Parker | Royal College of Surgeons of England |
| Mr D Mitchell | Faculty of Dental Surgery, Royal College of Surgeons of England |
| Dr M Osborn | Royal College of Pathologists |
| Ms S Panizzo | Patient Representative |
| Mrs M Wang | Patient Representative |

***Observers***

| | |
|---|---|
| Mrs C Miles | Institute of Healthcare Management |
| Dr R Hunter | Coroners' Society of England and Wales |
| Dr N Pace | Scottish Audit of Surgical Mortality |
| Professor P Littlejohns | National Institute for Health and Clinical Excellence |

NCEPOD is a company, limited by guarantee (Company number: 3019382) and a registered charity (Charity number: 1075588), managed by Trustees.

### *Trustees*



### *Clinical Co-ordinators*

The Steering Group appoint a Lead Clinical Co-ordinator for a defined tenure. In addition there are seven Clinical Co-ordinators who work on each study. All Co-ordinators are engaged in active academic/clinical practice (in the NHS) during their term of office.

Lead Clinical Co-ordinator

| | |
|---|---|
| Dr G Findlay | (Intensive Care) |

Clinical Co-ordinators

| | |
|---|---|
| Dr J A D Stewart | (Medicine) |
| Dr D G Mason | (Anaesthesia) |
| Dr K Wilkinson | (Anaesthesia) |
| Dr A P L Goodwin | (Anaesthesia) |
| Professor S B Lucas | (Pathology) |
| Mr I C Martin | (Surgery) |
| Professor M J Gough | (Surgery) |

### *Supporting organisations*

The organisations that provided funding to cover the cost of this study:
National Patient Safety Agency on behalf of the Department of Health in England and the Welsh Assembly Government
Department of Health, Social Services and Public Safety (Northern Ireland)
Aspen Healthcare Ltd
BMI Healthcare
BUPA Cromwell
Classic Hospitals
Covenant Healthcare Ltd
East Kent Medical Services Ltd
Fairfield Independent Hospital
HCA International
Hospital of St John and St Elizabeth
Isle of Man Health and Social Security Department
King Edward VII's Hospital Sister Agnes
Netcare Healthcare UK Ltd
New Victoria Hospital
Nuffield Health
Ramsay Health Care UK
Spire Health Care
St Anthony's Hospital
St Joseph's Hospital
States of Guernsey Board of Health
States of Jersey, Health and Social Services
The Benenden Hospital Trust
The Horder Centre
The Hospital Management Trust
The London Clinic
The London Oncology Clinic
Ulster Independent Clinic

# Appendix 4

## Trust participation

| Trust | Number of sites participating | Number of organisational questionnaire received | Number of included cases | Number of surgical questionnaires received | Number of cases in which notified of reason for null return of surgical questionnaires | Number of anaesthetic questionnaires received | Number of cases in which notified of reason for null return of Anaesthetic questionnaires | Number of cases in which the anaesthetic questionnaire was not applicable | Number of sets of case notes received | Number of cases in which the Trust was unable to retrieve case |
|---|---|---|---|---|---|---|---|---|---|---|
| Abertawe Bro Morgannwg University Health Board | 4 | 0* | 28 | 4 | 0 | 1 | 0 | 2 | 0 | |
| Aintree Hospitals NHS Foundation Trust | 1 | 1 | 22 | 13 | 2 | 11 | 8 | 2 | 10 | |
| Airedale NHS Trust | 1 | 1 | 8 | 7 | 1 | 6 | 0 | 0 | 4 | |
| Aneurin Bevan Local Health Board | 4 | 3 | 27 | 7 | 8 | 10 | 3 | 6 | 3 | 2 |
| Ashford & St Peter's Hospital NHS Trust | 2 | 2 | 2 | 2 | 0 | 0 | 0 | 1 | 2 | |
| Aspen Healthcare | 1 | 1 | 1 | 1 | 0 | 0 | 1 | 0 | 0 | |
| Barking, Havering & Redbridge University Hospitals NHS Trust | 2 | 2 | 20 | 15 | 3 | 10 | 3 | 6 | 17 | 1 |
| Barnet and Chase Farm Hospitals NHS Trust | 2 | 2 | 21 | 12 | 3 | 10 | 2 | 1 | 6 | |
| Barnsley Hospital NHS Foundation Trust | 1 | 0 | 5 | 3 | 2 | 4 | 0 | 1 | 1 | |
| Barts and The London NHS Trust | 3 | 2 | 13 | 2 | 2 | 1 | 2 | 0 | 1 | |
| Basildon & Thurrock University Hospitals NHS FoundationTrust | 1 | 1 | 24 | 18 | 1 | 13 | 4 | 4 | 8 | |
| Bedford Hospital NHS Trust | 1 | 1 | 9 | 9 | 0 | 5 | 3 | 0 | 9 | |
| Belfast Health and Social Care Trust | 3 | 3 | 13 | 4 | 2 | 7 | 0 | 3 | 5 | |
| Betsi Cadwaladr University Local Health Board | 3 | 2 | 7 | 6 | 1 | 4 | 0 | 1 | 2 | |
| Birmingham Women's Healthcare NHS Trust | 1 | 1 | 0 | 0 | 0 | 0 | 0 | 0 | 0 | |
| Blackpool, Fylde and Wyre Hospitals NHS Foundation Trust | 1 | 1 | 10 | 8 | 1 | 8 | 0 | 0 | 3 | |
| BMI Healthcare | 20 | 15 | 0 | 0 | 0 | 0 | 0 | 0 | 0 | |
| Bradford Teaching Hospitals NHS Foundation Trust | 1 | 1 | 9 | 5 | 0 | 4 | 4 | 1 | 4 | |

| | | | | | | | | | | |
|---|---|---|---|---|---|---|---|---|---|---|
| Brighton and Sussex University Hospitals NHS Trust | 3 | 1 | 16 | 10 | 1 | 6 | 3 | 0 | 10 | |
| Buckinghamshire Hospitals NHS Trust | 2 | 2 | 12 | 12 | 0 | 11 | 0 | 1 | 12 | |
| BUPA Cromwell Hospital | 1 | 0 | 0 | 0 | 0 | 0 | 0 | 0 | 0 | |
| Burton Hospitals NHS Foundation Trust | 1 | 1 | 5 | 4 | 1 | 5 | 0 | 0 | 5 | |
| Calderdale & Huddersfield NHS Foundation Trust | 2 | 2 | 13 | 11 | 2 | 8 | 3 | 1 | 11 | |
| Cambridge University Hospitals NHS Foundation Trust | 1 | 1 | 2 | 0 | 1 | 0 | 0 | 0 | 0 | |
| Cambridgeshire Community Services | 1 | 0 | 0 | 0 | 0 | 0 | 0 | 0 | 0 | |
| Cardiff and Vale University Local Health Board | 3 | 2 | 13 | 8 | 2 | 8 | 5 | 0 | 5 | 1 |
| Central Manchester University Hospitals NHS Foundation Trust | 4 | 0 | 10 | 5 | 1 | 4 | 3 | 2 | 1 | |
| Chelsea & Westminster Healthcare NHS Trust | 1 | 1 | 4 | 3 | 0 | 0 | 0 | 1 | 2 | |
| Chesterfield Royal Hospital NHS Foundation Trust | 1 | 1 | 11 | 9 | 0 | 10 | 0 | 0 | 7 | |
| City Hospitals Sunderland NHS Foundation Trust | 1 | 1 | 10 | 8 | 0 | 10 | 0 | 0 | 8 | |
| Colchester Hospital University NHS Foundation Trust | 2 | 2 | 15 | 7 | 5 | 6 | 2 | 0 | 6 | 2 |
| Countess of Chester Hospital NHS Foundation Trust | 1 | 1 | 0 | 0 | 0 | 0 | 0 | 0 | 0 | |
| County Durham and Darlington NHS Foundation Trust | 3 | 0 | 19 | 8 | 3 | 8 | 8 | 2 | 3 | 1 |
| Covenant Healthcare Limited | 2 | 2 | 0 | 0 | 0 | 0 | 0 | 0 | 0 | |
| Derby Hospitals NHS Foundation Trust | 2 | 1 | 8 | 6 | 2 | 7 | 1 | 0 | 8 | |
| Doncaster and Bassetlaw Hospitals NHS Foundation Trust | 3 | 3 | 13 | 8 | 2 | 5 | 2 | 3 | 2 | 1 |
| Dorset County Hospital NHS Foundation Trust | 1 | 1 | 4 | 4 | 0 | 4 | 0 | 0 | 4 | |
| Dudley Group of Hospitals NHS Trust | 1 | 1 | 16 | 14 | 1 | 4 | 2 | 6 | 6 | |
| Ealing Hospital NHS Trust | 1 | 1 | 1 | 0 | 0 | 1 | 0 | 0 | 0 | |
| East Cheshire NHS Trust | 1 | 1 | 7 | 4 | 2 | 4 | 1 | 1 | 2 | |

**Trust participation**
*(continued)*

| Trust | Number of sites participating | Number of organisational questionnaire received | Number of included cases | Number of surgical questionnaires received | Number of cases in which notified of reason for null return of surgical questionnaires | Number of anaesthetic questionnaires received | Number of cases in which notified of reason for null return of Anaesthetic questionnaires | Number of cases in which the anaesthetic questionnaire was not applicable | Number of sets of case notes received | Number of cases in which the Trust was unable to retrieve case |
|---|---|---|---|---|---|---|---|---|---|---|
| East Kent Hospitals University NHS Foundation Trust | 3 | 3 | 35 | 16 | 11 | 19 | 6 | 7 | 13 | 1 |
| East Lancashire Hospitals NHS Trust | 2 | 1 | 13 | 5 | 1 | 6 | 0 | 2 | 2 | |
| East Sussex Hospitals NHS Trust | 2 | 2 | 35 | 24 | 0 | 18 | 2 | 2 | 19 | |
| Epsom and St Helier University Hospitals NHS Trust | 3 | 1 | 14 | 7 | 3 | 1 | 1 | 0 | 5 | 1 |
| Frimley Park Hospitals NHS Trust | 1 | 1 | 6 | 6 | 0 | 5 | 0 | 1 | 4 | |
| Gateshead Health NHS Foundation Trust | 1 | 1 | 7 | 2 | 1 | 5 | 2 | 0 | 2 | |
| Great Western Hospitals NHS Foundation Trust | 1 | 1 | 5 | 5 | 0 | 3 | 0 | 2 | 5 | |
| Guy's & St Thomas' NHS Foundation Trust | 2 | 0 | 9 | 4 | 1 | 3 | 0 | 0 | 3 | |
| Harrogate and District NHS Foundation Trust | 1 | 1 | 7 | 6 | 1 | 6 | 0 | 1 | 7 | |
| HCA International | 2 | 1 | 2 | 2 | 0 | 2 | 0 | 0 | 2 | |
| Health & Social Services, States of Guernsey | 1 | 1 | 0 | 0 | 0 | 0 | 0 | 0 | 0 | |
| Heart of England NHS Foundation Trust | 3 | 0 | 12 | 9 | 1 | 5 | 2 | 1 | 3 | |
| Heatherwood & Wexham Park Hospitals NHS Foundation Trust | 2 | 0 | 16 | 10 | 1 | 4 | 1 | 1 | 2 | |
| Hereford Hospitals NHS Trust | 1 | 1 | 5 | 5 | 0 | 5 | 0 | 0 | 5 | |
| Hillingdon Hospital NHS Trust | 2 | 1 | 8 | 2 | 4 | 6 | 1 | 1 | 0 | |
| Hinchingbrooke Health Care NHS Trust | 1 | 1 | 7 | 6 | 1 | 3 | 2 | 1 | 5 | |
| Homerton University Hospital NHS Foundation Trust | 1 | 1 | 6 | 5 | 0 | 5 | 0 | 1 | 2 | |

| | | | | | | | | | | |
|---|---|---|---|---|---|---|---|---|---|---|
| Hospital of St John and St Elizabeth | 1 | 1 | 1 | 0 | 0 | 0 | 0 | 0 | 0 | |
| Hull and East Yorkshire Hospitals NHS Trust | 3 | 2 | 13 | 11 | 1 | 8 | 2 | 3 | 11 | |
| Hywel Dda Local Health Board | 4 | 3 | 13 | 6 | 1 | 7 | 2 | 0 | 2 | 1 |
| Imperial College Healthcare NHS Trust | 4 | 4 | 14 | 11 | 0 | 11 | 0 | 0 | 10 | |
| Ipswich Hospital NHS Trust | 1 | 0 | 14 | 10 | 2 | 12 | 1 | 1 | 7 | |
| Isle of Man Department of Health & Social Security | 1 | 0 | 1 | 1 | 0 | 1 | 0 | 0 | 1 | |
| Isle of Wight NHS Primary Care Trust | 1 | 1 | 9 | 8 | 0 | 5 | 2 | 1 | 7 | |
| James Paget Healthcare NHS Trust | 1 | 1 | 12 | 8 | 4 | 9 | 0 | 3 | 11 | |
| Kettering General Hospital NHS Trust | 1 | 0 | 0 | 0 | 0 | 0 | 0 | 0 | 0 | |
| King Edward VII's Hospital Sister Agnes | 1 | 1 | 0 | 0 | 0 | 0 | 0 | 0 | 0 | |
| King's College Hospital NHS Foundation Trust | 1 | 0 | 11 | 6 | 0 | 5 | 1 | 0 | 9 | |
| Kingston Hospital NHS Trust | 1 | 1 | 7 | 5 | 0 | 5 | 1 | 0 | 3 | |
| Lancashire Teaching Hospitals NHS Foundation Trust | 2 | 2 | 26 | 9 | 1 | 2 | 1 | 0 | 5 | |
| Leeds Teaching Hospitals NHS Trust (The) | 5 | 5 | 15 | 7 | 3 | 5 | 6 | 0 | 5 | 1 |
| Lewisham Hospital NHS Trust | 1 | 1 | 8 | 6 | 2 | 3 | 0 | 5 | 8 | |
| Liverpool Heart and Chest Hospital NHS Trust | 1 | 0 | 3 | 2 | 0 | 1 | 0 | 0 | 2 | |
| Liverpool Women's NHS Foundation Trust | 1 | 1 | 1 | 1 | 0 | 1 | 0 | 0 | 1 | |
| London Clinic | 1 | 1 | 0 | 0 | 0 | 0 | 0 | 0 | 0 | |
| Luton and Dunstable Hospital NHS Foundation Trust | 1 | 1 | 6 | 4 | 0 | 1 | 1 | 0 | 3 | |
| Maidstone and Tunbridge Wells NHS Trust | 3 | 2 | 18 | 15 | 1 | 5 | 3 | 0 | 8 | 1 |
| Mayday Health Care NHS Trust | 1 | 1 | 7 | 2 | 1 | 2 | 3 | 0 | 1 | |
| Mid Cheshire Hospitals NHS Trust | 2 | 1 | 7 | 2 | 1 | 4 | 1 | 1 | 2 | |
| Mid Staffordshire NHS Foundation Trust | 2 | 2 | 9 | 7 | 2 | 2 | 6 | 1 | 4 | 1 |
| Mid Yorkshire Hospitals NHS Trust | 4 | 4 | 18 | 13 | 2 | 6 | 5 | 1 | 17 | |
| Mid-Essex Hospital Services NHS Trust | 1 | 1 | 14 | 9 | 1 | 10 | 0 | 2 | 8 | |
| Milton Keynes Hospital NHS Foundation Trust | 1 | 1 | 7 | 0 | 5 | 5 | 0 | 1 | 2 | |
| Moorfields Eye Hospital NHS Foundation Trust | 1 | 0 | 0 | 0 | 0 | 0 | 0 | 0 | 0 | |

**Trust participation**
*(continued)*

| Trust | Number of sites participating | Number of organisational questionnaire received | Number of included cases | Number of surgical questionnaires received | Number of cases in which notified of reason for null return of surgical questionnaires | Number of anaesthetic questionnaires received | Number of cases in which notified of reason for null return of Anaesthetic questionnaires | Number of cases in which the anaesthetic questionnaire was not applicable | Number of sets of case notes received | Number of cases in which the Trust was unable to retrieve case |
|---|---|---|---|---|---|---|---|---|---|---|
| New Victoria Hospital | 1 | 1 | 0 | 0 | 0 | 0 | 0 | 0 | 0 | |
| Newcastle upon Tyne Hospitals NHS Foundation Trust | 3 | 3 | 14 | 12 | 1 | 10 | 1 | 1 | 10 | |
| Newham University Hospital NHS Trust | 1 | 0 | 1 | 0 | 0 | 0 | 0 | 0 | 0 | |
| Norfolk & Norwich University Hospital NHS Trust | 2 | 2 | 22 | 14 | 3 | 12 | 3 | 5 | 9 | |
| North Bristol NHS Trust | 2 | 1 | 23 | 16 | 3 | 14 | 5 | 3 | 15 | 2 |
| North Cumbria Acute Hospitals NHS Trust | 2 | 0 | 14 | 0 | 0 | 0 | 0 | 0 | 0 | |
| North Middlesex University Hospital NHS Trust | 1 | 1 | 3 | 3 | 0 | 1 | 1 | 0 | 1 | |
| North Tees and Hartlepool NHS Foundation Trust | 2 | 2 | 7 | 3 | 0 | 3 | 0 | 0 | 2 | |
| North West London Hospitals NHS Trust | 3 | 3 | 10 | 10 | 0 | 9 | 0 | 1 | 10 | |
| Northampton General Hospital NHS Trust | 1 | 1 | 10 | 6 | 2 | 4 | 5 | 0 | 6 | 1 |
| Northern Devon Healthcare NHS Trust | 1 | 1 | 5 | 3 | 1 | 2 | 2 | 1 | 4 | |
| Northern Health & Social CareTrust | 1 | 1 | 0 | 0 | 0 | 0 | 0 | 0 | 0 | |
| Northern Lincolnshire & Goole Hospitals NHS Foundation Trust | 3 | 2 | 6 | 4 | 0 | 5 | 0 | 1 | 0 | |
| Northumbria Healthcare NHS Foundation Trust | 6 | 2 | 15 | 12 | 0 | 12 | 1 | 1 | 6 | |
| Nottingham University Hospitals NHS Trust | 2 | 2 | 20 | 13 | 2 | 14 | 1 | 0 | 7 | |
| Nuffield Health | 15 | 11 | 0 | 0 | 0 | 0 | 0 | 0 | 0 | |
| Nuffield Orthopaedic Centre NHS Trust | 1 | 1 | 2 | 1 | 0 | 1 | 0 | 1 | 0 | |

| | | | | | | | | | | |
|---|---|---|---|---|---|---|---|---|---|---|
| Oxford Radcliffe Hospital NHS Trust | 3 | 3 | 37 | 32 | 3 | 23 | 8 | 4 | 35 | |
| Papworth Hospital NHS Foundation Trust | 1 | 1 | 2 | 2 | 0 | 1 | 0 | 1 | 2 | |
| Pennine Acute Hospitals NHS Trust (The) | 4 | 4 | 26 | 11 | 5 | 21 | 2 | 0 | 18 | 1 |
| Peterborough & Stamford Hospitals NHS Foundation Trust | 3 | 3 | 7 | 5 | 1 | 6 | 1 | 0 | 4 | 1 |
| Plymouth Hospitals NHS Trust | 2 | 1 | 14 | 13 | 1 | 13 | 1 | 0 | 14 | |
| Poole Hospital NHS Foundation Trust | 1 | 1 | 14 | 11 | 1 | 11 | 3 | 0 | 3 | |
| Portsmouth Hospitals NHS Trust | 2 | 1 | 22 | 7 | 10 | 8 | 8 | 1 | 5 | 4 |
| Powys Teaching Local Health Board | 2 | 2 | 0 | 0 | 0 | 0 | 0 | 0 | 0 | |
| Princess Alexandra Hospital NHS Trust | 2 | 1 | 10 | 8 | 0 | 2 | 0 | 1 | 4 | |
| Queen Victoria Hospital NHS Foundation Trust | 1 | 1 | 1 | 1 | 0 | 1 | 0 | 0 | 1 | |
| Ramsay Health Care UK | 19 | 17 | 1 | 1 | 0 | 0 | 1 | 0 | 1 | |
| Royal Berkshire NHS Foundation Trust | 1 | 1 | 13 | 12 | 0 | 12 | 0 | 1 | 5 | |
| Royal Bolton Hospital NHS Foundation Trust | 1 | 1 | 10 | 8 | 0 | 5 | 0 | 1 | 5 | |
| Royal Bournemouth and Christchurch Hospitals NHS Trust | 2 | 2 | 9 | 8 | 1 | 6 | 1 | 2 | 8 | |
| Royal Brompton and Harefield NHS Trust | 2 | 2 | 4 | 4 | 0 | 4 | 0 | 0 | 4 | |
| Royal Cornwall Hospitals NHS Trust | 3 | 3 | 10 | 9 | 1 | 10 | 0 | 0 | 10 | |
| Royal Devon and Exeter NHS Foundation Trust | 1 | 1 | 16 | 16 | 0 | 13 | 0 | 3 | 16 | |
| Royal Free Hampstead NHS Trust | 2 | 2 | 3 | 3 | 0 | 2 | 0 | 1 | 3 | |
| Royal Liverpool & Broadgreen University Hospitals NHS Trust | 2 | 1 | 11 | 11 | 0 | 8 | 1 | 2 | 11 | |
| Royal Marsden NHS Foundation Trust (The) | 2 | 1 | 0 | 0 | 0 | 0 | 0 | 0 | 0 | |
| Royal National Orthopaedic Hospital NHS Trust | 1 | 1 | 0 | 0 | 0 | 0 | 0 | 0 | 0 | |
| Royal Orthopaedic Hospital NHS Foundation Trust | 1 | 1 | 0 | 0 | 0 | 0 | 0 | 0 | 0 | |
| Royal Surrey County Hospital NHS Trust | 1 | 1 | 6 | 5 | 1 | 4 | 2 | 0 | 5 | |
| Royal United Hospital Bath NHS Trust | 1 | 1 | 17 | 15 | 2 | 15 | 2 | 0 | 15 | 2 |
| Salford Royal Hospitals NHS Foundation Trust | 1 | 1 | 7 | 3 | 0 | 6 | 0 | 0 | 0 | |
| Salisbury NHS Foundation Trust | 1 | 1 | 4 | 4 | 0 | 4 | 0 | 0 | 4 | |

## Trust participation
*(continued)*

| Trust | Number of sites participating | Number of organisational questionnaire received | Number of included cases | Number of surgical questionnaires received | Number of cases in which notified of reason for null return of surgical questionnaires | Number of anaesthetic questionnaires received | Number of cases in which notified of reason for null return of Anaesthetic questionnaires | Number of cases in which the anaesthetic questionnaire was not applicable | Number of sets of case notes received | Number of cases in which the Trust was unable to retrieve case |
|---|---|---|---|---|---|---|---|---|---|---|
| Sandwell and West Birmingham Hospitals NHS Trust | 2 | 2 | 16 | 11 | 2 | 10 | 1 | 2 | 14 | |
| Sheffield Teaching Hospitals NHS Foundation Trust | 3 | 1 | 31 | 22 | 7 | 22 | 8 | 1 | 24 | 4 |
| Sherwood Forest Hospitals NHS Trust | 3 | 2 | 15 | 13 | 0 | 7 | 1 | 3 | 15 | |
| Shrewsbury and Telford Hospitals NHS Trust | 2 | 1 | 8 | 6 | 1 | 3 | 0 | 2 | 6 | |
| Shropshire County Primary Care Trust | 1 | 1 | 0 | 0 | 0 | 0 | 0 | 0 | 0 | |
| South Devon Healthcare NHS Foundation Trust | 1 | 1 | 12 | 8 | 3 | 8 | 3 | 0 | 3 | |
| South Eastern Health & Social Care Trust | 3 | 3 | 8 | 5 | 0 | 3 | 1 | 0 | 3 | |
| South London Healthcare NHS Trust | 3 | 2 | 22 | 13 | 5 | 15 | 5 | 0 | 7 | |
| South Tees Hospitals NHS Foundation Trust | 2 | 2 | 10 | 10 | 0 | 5 | 3 | 1 | 6 | |
| South Tyneside NHS Foundation Trust | 1 | 1 | 0 | 0 | 0 | 0 | 0 | 0 | 0 | |
| South Warwickshire General Hospitals NHS Trust | 1 | 1 | 10 | 10 | 0 | 4 | 3 | 1 | 0 | |
| Southampton University Hospitals NHS Trust | 1 | 0 | 35 | 22 | 1 | 9 | 0 | 2 | 21 | |
| Southend University Hospital NHS Foundation Trust | 1 | 0 | 23 | 8 | 5 | 14 | 2 | 1 | 5 | |
| Southport and Ormskirk Hospitals NHS Trust | 1 | 1 | 6 | 5 | 1 | 2 | 3 | 1 | 1 | |
| Spire Healthcare | 16 | 14 | 1 | 1 | 0 | 0 | 0 | 0 | 1 | |
| St Anthony's Hospital | 1 | 1 | 1 | 1 | 0 | 1 | 0 | 0 | 1 | |
| St George's Healthcare NHS Trust | 1 | 0 | 18 | 8 | 2 | 6 | 3 | 0 | 3 | 2 |

| St Helens and Knowsley Teaching Hospitals NHS Trust | 2 | 2 | 12 | 12 | 0 | 12 | 0 | 0 | 12 | |
|---|---|---|---|---|---|---|---|---|---|---|
| Surrey & Sussex Healthcare NHS Trust | 1 | 1 | 15 | 14 | 0 | 13 | 0 | 0 | 14 | |
| Taunton & Somerset NHS Foundation Trust | 1 | 1 | 9 | 9 | 0 | 7 | 1 | 1 | 9 | |
| The Hospital Management Trust | 2 | 2 | 0 | 0 | 0 | 0 | 0 | 0 | 0 | |
| The Queen Elizabeth Hospital King's Lynn NHS Trust | 1 | 1 | 0 | 0 | 0 | 0 | 0 | 0 | 0 | |
| The Rotherham NHS Foundation Trust | 1 | 1 | 6 | 4 | 2 | 3 | 2 | 1 | 6 | |
| United Lincolnshire Hospitals NHS Trust | 4 | 4 | 19 | 12 | 0 | 13 | 1 | 0 | 1 | |
| Univ. Hospital of South Manchester NHS Foundation Trust | 1 | 1 | 14 | 8 | 0 | 7 | 1 | 4 | 6 | |
| University College London Hospitals NHS Foundation Trust | 4 | 3 | 8 | 3 | 5 | 4 | 1 | 0 | 6 | |
| University Hospital Birmingham NHS Foundation Trust | 2 | 2 | 7 | 7 | 0 | 3 | 0 | 1 | 7 | |
| University Hospitals Coventry and Warwickshire NHS Trust | 2 | 2 | 21 | 15 | 6 | 19 | 0 | 2 | 21 | |
| University Hospitals of Bristol NHS Foundation Trust | 4 | 4 | 14 | 7 | 5 | 10 | 3 | 0 | 4 | |
| University Hospitals of Leicester NHS Trust | 3 | 3 | 2 | 2 | 0 | 1 | 1 | 0 | 2 | |
| University Hospitals of Morecambe Bay NHS Trust | 3 | 0 | 21 | 11 | 3 | 15 | 1 | 2 | 17 | 1 |
| Walsall Hospitals NHS Trust | 1 | 0 | 15 | 10 | 4 | 11 | 2 | 0 | 2 | |
| Warrington & Halton Hospitals NHS Foundation Trust | 2 | 1 | 18 | 11 | 4 | 7 | 2 | 3 | 3 | 1 |
| West Middlesex University Hospital NHS Trust | 1 | 1 | 8 | 4 | 0 | 7 | 0 | 1 | 2 | |
| West Suffolk Hospitals NHS Trust | 1 | 1 | 7 | 6 | 1 | 6 | 0 | 0 | 7 | |
| Western Health & Social Care Trust | 1 | 1 | 5 | 2 | 2 | 3 | 0 | 0 | 2 | |
| Western Sussex Hospitals NHS Trust | 3 | 2 | 21 | 10 | 1 | 9 | 1 | 2 | 10 | |
| Weston Area Health Trust | 1 | 0 | 6 | 4 | 0 | 3 | 1 | 2 | 4 | |
| Whipps Cross University Hospital NHS Trust | 1 | 1 | 11 | 6 | 3 | 4 | 5 | 0 | 2 | 2 |
| Whittington Hospital NHS Trust | 1 | 1 | 4 | 3 | 1 | 2 | 1 | 1 | 2 | 1 |

**Trust participation**
*(continued)*

| | Number of sites participating | Number of organisational questionnaire received | Number of included cases | Number of surgical questionnaires received | Number of cases in which notified of reason for null return of surgical questionnaires | Number of anaesthetic questionnaires received | Number of cases in which notified of reason for null return of Anaesthetic questionnaires | Number of cases in which the anaesthetic questionnaire was not applicable | Number of sets of case notes received | Number of cases in which the Trust was unable to retrieve case |
|---|---|---|---|---|---|---|---|---|---|---|
| Winchester & Eastleigh Healthcare NHS Trust | 1 | 1 | 11 | 9 | 0 | 6 | 3 | 0 | 1 | |
| Wirral University Teaching Hospital | | | | | | | | | | |
| NHS Foundation Trust | 2 | 1 | 21 | 7 | 2 | 6 | 2 | 3 | 9 | |
| Worcestershire Acute Hospitals | 2 | 2 | 20 | 16 | 0 | 14 | 2 | 0 | 7 | |
| Wrightington, Wigan & Leigh | | | | | | | | | | |
| NHS Foundation Trust | 3 | 3 | 11 | 6 | 3 | 6 | 3 | 2 | 8 | |
| Yeovil District Hospital | | | | | | | | | | |
| NHS Foundation Trust | 1 | 1 | 6 | 2 | 1 | 1 | 1 | 3 | 5 | |
| York Hospitals NHS Foundation Trust | 1 | 1 | 13 | 11 | 2 | 8 | 2 | 3 | 7 | |

*Notification of participation in the study was too late for organisational questionnaires to be sent out and included in the study.

Trusts/hospitals from which no data was received and for which no reason was provided:

**Basingstoke & North Hampshire Hospitals NHS Foundation Trust**
**Benenden Hospital**
**Cwm Taf Local Health Board**
**Dartford & Gravesham NHS Trust**
**East & North Hertfordshire NHS Trust**
**George Eliot Hospital NHS Trust**
**Gloucestershire Hospitals NHS Foundation Trust**
**HCA International**
**Medway NHS Foundation Trust**
**Northern Health & Social CareTrust**
**Royal Wolverhampton Hospitals NHS Trust (The)**
**Scarborough and North East Yorkshire Health Care NHS Trust**
**Southern Health & Social Care Trust**
**States of Jersey Health & Social Services**
**Stockport NHS Foundation Trust**
**Tameside Hospital NHS Foundation Trust**
**The Walton Centre NHS Foundation Trust**
**Trafford Healthcare NHS Trust**
**University Hospital of North Staffordshire NHS Trust**
**West Hertfordshire Hospitals NHS Trust**